POCKET
clinical
examination
3RD EDITION

POCKET

clinical examination

3RD EDITION

Nicholas J. Talley

MBBS (Hons, NSW), MMSci (Clin Epid) (Newcastle), MD (NSW), PhD (Syd),
FRACP, FRCP (London & Edinburgh), FAFPHM, FACP, FACG, AGAF
Professor of Medicine and Epidemiology, Mayo Clinic College of Medicine
Chair, Department of Internal Medicine, Mayo Clinic, Jacksonville
Consultant, Division of Gastroenterology & Hepatology, Mayo Clinic,
Jacksonville and Rochester
Visiting Professor, Department of Medicine, University of Sydney and
Nepean Hospital, Penrith, NSW

Simon O'Connor

MBBS (Syd), FRACP, DDU, FCSANZ
Cardiologist, The Canberra Hospital
Clinical Senior Lecturer, Australian National University Medical School,
Canberra, ACT

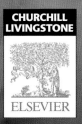

CHURCHILL
LIVINGSTONE

ELSEVIER

Sydney   Edinburgh   London   New York   Philadelphia   St Louis   Toronto

Churchill Livingstone
is an imprint of Elsevier

Elsevier Australia. ACN 001 002 357
(a division of Reed International Books Australia Pty Ltd)
Tower 1, 475 Victoria Avenue, Chatswood, NSW 2067

ELSEVIER

National Library of Australia Cataloguing-in-Publication Data

Talley, Nicholas Joseph.

Pocket clinical examination / Nicholas J Talley ; Simon O'Connor.

3rd ed

ISBN: 978 0 7295 3872 5 (pbk.)

Includes index.
Bibliography.

Physical diagnosis–Handbooks, manuals, etc.
Diagnosis–Handbooks, manuals, etc.

O'Connor, Simon.

616.0754

Publisher: Sophie Kaliniecki
Developmental Editor: Sunalie Silva
Publishing Services Manager: Helena Klijn
Editorial Coordinator: Lauren Allsop
Edited by Caroline Hunter, Burrumundi Pty Ltd
Proofread by Tim Learner
Illustrations by Joseph Lucia and TNQ Books & Journals Pvt. Ltd.
Cover, internal design and typesetting by DiZign Pty Ltd
Index by Max McMaster
Printed in China by 1010 Printing International Ltd

Contents

Foreword

Most aspiring physicians in Australia in the 1980s, preparing for a clinical examination involving long and short cases, trained by developing their own approaches to the majority of clinical exam scenarios. These approaches were honed with colleagues and remain with them today as they go about their clinical practice.

Nick Talley and Simon O'Connor have assembled their approaches into their now-famous textbooks, and this pocket version of clinical skills is now in its third edition. It has become an international best seller and a valuable companion for medical students, young physicians and clinicians who aspire to excellence in the art of medicine.

The book is probably best used as a basis for the development of your own approach to examination and history taking. Embellish, refine and modify the approaches suggested and your exams will become your own unique way of confirming clinical suspicions. When you think that you have a better way of examining a particular organ or system, contact the authors via the publisher with your suggestion. You too will then have made a contribution to the way others think and approach the art of medicine.

This is a valuable text that should inspire excellence.

Professor Bruce Robinson
Dean, Faculty of Medicine, University of Sydney

Preface

Physical Examination is ordinarily taken to mean examination of the patient using the examiner's five senses aided only by the portable tools of his trade such as stethoscope, tendon hammer, ophthalmoscope etc …

The Oxford Medical Companion (1994)

This third edition of *Pocket Clinical Examination* has been prepared as a companion to our major textbook, *Clinical Examination: A Systematic Guide to Physical Diagnosis*. A number of new chapters have been added to this edition, covering essential skills such as advanced history taking, assessment of the acutely ill patient, special aspects of the assessment of the geriatric patient and an introduction to examination of the skin. We have also included key anatomical drawings to assist you to understand the relevant clinical anatomy of the regions of the body you are learning to examine. In addition, hints on how to approach the Objective Structured Clinical Examinations (OSCEs), which most students have to face, are included.

With the preparation of this new edition has come the opportunity to update the book with an emphasis on evidence. The science of evidence-based medicine has come rather late to the field of physical examination, but it is now beginning to help guide the identification and teaching of essential clinical skills. See our textbook *Clinical Examination* for more details.

Although medical imaging and investigations are becoming increasingly sophisticated, in about 80% of cases the diagnosis of a medical condition is made, or strongly suspected, on the basis of the history and examination. The easy availability of various tests should not displace the careful clinical assessment of the patient. Tests ordered for the wrong reasons, because the patient has not been properly assessed, are often useless—or worse, dangerous.

We hope you enjoy this introduction to clinical skills, and that the knowledge imparted herein will prove valuable throughout your career. In the twenty-first century the delivery of medicine is optimally conducted as a team effort, and we all need to continue to learn from each other. Please contact us via the publisher if you have any suggestions or ideas for the next edition.

Nicholas J. Talley
Simon O'Connor
Jacksonville and Canberra
December 2008

Reviewers

Dr Ben Gupta BMedSci, BM, BS
Anaesthetic Registrar, Torbay Hospital, UK

Dr Anna Vnuk MBBS, DRACOG, FRACGP, Grad Cert Tert Ed, MClinEd
Director, Clinical Skills Lab and Senior Lecturer, Health Professional
Education, Clinical Skills and Simulation Unit, School of Medicine,
Flinders University

Dr Ashley Watson MBBS, Grad Cert Ed Stud, MPH, FRACP
Senior Specialist, Infectious Diseases Unit, The Canberra Hospital;
Associate Professor, ANU Medical School; and Chair, Clinical Skills,
ANUMS

chapter 1

Taking the history

The distance doesn't matter; it is only the first step that is difficult.

Marquise Du Deffand (1697–1780)

This is arguably the most important chapter that you'll read in medical school. Even in the twenty-first century, with all the rapid and exciting advances in biology, excellent history taking remains absolutely central to the best practice of medicine. Practising medicine remains an art and a science; here you will begin to learn how to acquire the necessary skills, which with practice should become second nature.

The history

As a doctor, you have a fundamental duty to understand your patients' stories. To help and to heal, you need to learn what your patients have experienced and what they feel. While every story is unique, doctors can deduce a reasonable diagnosis in most cases by listening carefully and asking the right questions. By narrowing the differential diagnosis (a list of the possible diagnoses suggested by a set of symptoms or signs), appropriate testing and therapy can be ordered.

Remember that *symptoms* are subjective feelings perceptible to the patient, while *signs* are changes that can be demonstrated objectively. Even if the possible diagnoses are not clear after the history has been taken, the probable region or system of the body that is affected will usually be obvious. This enables you to direct the examination and diagnostic tests appropriately.

Unless patients are extremely ill, the taking of a careful medical history should precede both examination and treatment. Taking the history and examining the patient are also, of course, the least expensive ways of making a diagnosis. *A good history will usually take you 80% of the way to making the right diagnosis.*

Bedside manner

The word 'clinical' is derived from the Greek word klīnikós, meaning 'of or pertaining to a bed' (*Oxford English Dictionary*, 2nd edn). The term 'bedside manner' describes the clinician's approach to the patient. A professional manner will make history taking and physical examination enjoyable and rewarding for both the student doctor and the patient. This is not an easy skill to describe or teach, but it should be learned at the bedside by observing the methods (both successful and unsuccessful) of senior colleagues.

At the end of the medical interview and examination the clinician must explain as clearly as possible to the patient what the clinical diagnosis is and what it means. The explanation must include discussion of the prognosis (the likely outcome of the illness) and the investigations, treatment and, if relevant, the probable length of hospital stay that are to be recommended to the patient.

Remember that the clinician's recommendations are just that; it should be clear to patients that they can freely accept or reject the recommendations (except in the most unusual circumstances). Good history taking improves the accuracy and completeness of the medical diagnosis and promotes the doctor–patient relationship.

Obtaining the history

The medical interview deals not only with the organic problems of the patient but also with any psychosocial aspects of the illness; the mind and body are not separate entities. In order to develop an effective interviewing technique, you must make a conscious effort to listen to the patient and to establish rapport.

It is useful to make rough notes while questioning the patient. At the end of the history taking and examination a detailed record is made. This record must be a *sequential*, accurate account of the development and course of the patient's illness or illnesses (even if this is not the order in which the questions were asked). A systematic approach to history taking and recording is the most reliable way to avoid missing crucial information (see Table 1.1). At the end, the record must make it clear whether the patient's problem is one of diagnosis (i.e. what is wrong) or of management (i.e. what tests and treatment are necessary), or both.

Introductory questions

Introduce yourself to the patient. It is important here to address the patient respectfully and to use his or her name and title. It is usually sufficient to introduce yourself to the patient as a student doctor.

In order to obtain a good history, you must interview in a **logical manner**, **listen** carefully, **interrupt** appropriately (focusing on encouraging the patient to tell the full story in his or her own words first), note **non-verbal clues**, establish a **good relationship** and **correctly interpret** the information obtained.

Table 1.1 History-taking documentation
Presenting (principal) symptom (PS)
History of presenting illness (HPI) Details of current symptoms or complaints Details of previous similar episodes Current and recent treatment (all drugs: doses, duration, indication) Extent of functional disability
Past history (PH) Past illnesses Past surgical operations (dates and indications) Past treatments Blood transfusions Drug allergies Health maintenance (disease prevention) Menstrual and reproductive history for women
Social history (SH) Occupation, education, place of birth Marital status, social support, living conditions Smoking history and alcohol consumption Use of analgesics Overseas travel Sexual and drug abuse history
Family history (FH) Diseases in first-degree relatives
Systems review (SR)

You should sit down beside the patient so as to be close to eye level and give the impression that the interview will be an unhurried one. The next step should be to **find out the patient's major complaint or complaints**. It is best to attempt a conversational approach and ask 'What has been the trouble or problem recently?' or 'When did these problems begin?' If the patient has already been interviewed by the resident, the registrar, the consultant and three medical students, it may be necessary to apologise and explain the importance of hearing about the problem again in the patient's own words. **Allow the patient to tell the whole story, then ask questions to fill in the gaps**.

To ensure the best possible communication between the patient and doctor it is important to try to make the patient feel comfortable. Try to appear (and feel) relaxed and not in a hurry, even if it is lunchtime. Appropriate (but not exaggerated) reassuring gestures may be useful. If the patient stops telling the story spontaneously, it can be helpful to provide a short summary of what has already been said and then encourage the patient to continue.

Learn to listen with an open mind. The temptation to leap to specific questions before the patient has had the chance to describe all the symptoms in his or her own words should be resisted. However, some direction may be necessary to keep a talkative patient on track later during the interview. Avoid using pseudo-medical terms and, if the patient uses them, find out exactly what is meant by them, because misinterpretation of medical terms is common.

While the patient is describing the symptoms, make observations to help you draw inferences about the patient's personality. For example, note dress, facial expressions (e.g. the amount of distress while describing personal matters), signs of anxiety or restlessness and mannerisms as you discuss issues with the patient. Some patients may have medical problems that make the interview difficult for them; these include deafness and problems with speech and memory. These must be recognised if the interview is to be successful. For confused or forgetful patients, the history may have to be obtained partly or completely via a suitable family member or close friend.

It is suggested that the history be recorded and presented roughly in the order described below. However, open-ended questions often result in the information being obtained in a different sequence, so you will need to rearrange this information for recording and presentation.

The presenting (principal or chief) symptom (or complaint) (PS)

An attempt must be made to decide which of the patient's symptoms (there may be more than one) led the patient to present. It must be remembered that the patient's and the doctor's idea of what constitutes a serious problem may differ. Record each presenting symptom in the patient's own words, avoiding technical terms. Later on, the symptoms should be recorded in a more formal medical format.

Current symptoms and history of the presenting illness (HPI)

Let the patient describe the symptoms that have caused him or her to seek medical help. Quite a lot of detail about the course and nature of *all* the symptoms is required. When the history of the presenting illness is written down, the events should be placed in chronological order or, if numerous systems are affected, in chronological order for each system.

Certain information should routinely be sought for *each* of the symptoms if this hasn't been volunteered by the patient. The mnemonic SOCRATES summarises the questions that should be asked about most symptoms:

- **S**ite
- **O**nset
- **C**haracter and severity
- **R**adiation
- **A**ggravating and relieving factors
- **T**iming
- **E**xacerbating factors and associated symptoms
- **S**ocial aspects (effect of the symptom or illness).

Site
Ask where the symptom is exactly and whether it is **localised or diffuse**. Ask the patient to point to the actual site on the body. Also determine whether the symptom, if localised, radiates (travels elsewhere). Other symptoms, such as cough, dyspnoea (shortness of breath), change in weight or dizziness, are not localised.

Onset
Find out when the **symptom first began** and try to date this as accurately as possible. A patient asked 'How long has this pain been present?' will not uncommonly say, 'For a long time, doctor'. It is necessary then to ask 'Do you mean a few hours or many weeks?' Although you should not suggest answers to the patient, giving a few possible alternatives may speed up the process.

Character and severity
Ask the patient **what is meant by the symptom**. If the patient complains of dizziness, does this mean the room spins around (vertigo) or is it more a feeling of light-headedness? It may be necessary to suggest some alternative descriptions. For example, a patient may find chest discomfort difficult to describe. It is reasonable then to ask whether the feeling is tight, heavy, sharp or stabbing. It is interesting to note that patients who have been stabbed do not usually describe the pain as stabbing.

Symptom **severity** is subjective. The best way to assess severity is to ask the patient whether the symptom interferes with normal activities or sleep. It is useful to ask the patient to grade any pain by a number between 0 and 10, where 10 represents the most severe pain the patient has ever experienced and 0 represents no pain. Alternatively, you can ask whether pain, or other symptom, is mild, moderate, severe or very severe.

Radiation
The pattern of **radiation** is very suggestive of certain abnormalities—for example, the distribution of pain and paraesthesiae (pins and needles) in the territory of the median nerve of the hand in carpal tunnel syndrome.

Aggravating and relieving factors
Ask whether anything makes the symptom worse or better. For example, lying flat may make the dyspnoea of heart failure worse but not that of chronic obstructive pulmonary disease (chronic bronchitis or emphysema).

Timing
Find out whether the **symptom came on rapidly**, **gradually** or **instantaneously** at the date of onset. Certain symptoms are typically of very sudden onset (like turning on a light)—for example, the onset of a fast heartbeat in supraventricular tachycardia. Ask whether the symptom has been present continuously or intermittently. Determine whether the symptom is getting worse or better and, if so, when the change occurred.

Some symptoms are at their very worst at the moment of onset (e.g. the pain of an aortic tear called a dissection). Find out what the patient was doing at the time the symptom began.

Exacerbating factors and associated symptoms

Here an attempt is made to uncover in a systematic way symptoms that might be expected to be associated with a particular disease or **risk factors** that make a disease more likely. For example, a strong family history of carcinoma of the colon makes rectal bleeding a more sinister symptom. A patient who presents with cardiac symptoms must have the major risk factors for coronary artery disease (e.g. smoking and family history) assessed in detail.

Social aspects (impact of the symptom or illness)

Any serious or chronic illness may cause severe financial or social problems that should be explored and documented. These problems need to be taken into account when planning the best treatment.

Current treatment

Ask the patient whether he or she is currently taking any tablets or medicines. Attempt to find out the names and doses of each, and the reason for taking the medicine. Remember that non-prescription drugs and alternative therapies may not be thought relevant by the patient and may have to be asked about specifically. Always ask whether a woman is taking a contraceptive pill because it is not considered a medicine or tablet by many who take it.

Past history (PH)

Next, aspects of the patient's past history that have not yet emerged must be sought systematically.

Past illnesses and surgical operations

Ask the patient whether there have been any serious illnesses or operations or admissions to hospital in the past and at what age these occurred. For each surgery, ask about the indication. Find out about serious illnesses in childhood that interfered with school. It is often necessary to ask how a particular diagnosis was made in the past, as the patient's impression of what was wrong may not be correct.

A history of multiple accidents or serious illnesses may suggest another underlying problem. For example, alcohol or drug abuse may be the cause of repeated motor accidents or head injuries. Elderly patients may have multiple falls because of neurological or bone disease.

Past treatments

There are some medications or treatments the patient may have had in the past that remain relevant: these include corticosteroids, oral contraceptives, antihypertensive agents, blood transfusions, and chemotherapy or radiotherapy for malignancy. The thrombolytic drug streptokinase, for example, should not be readministered for at least a year because of antibody production and the risk of allergic reactions and ineffectiveness.

Drug allergies

Note any adverse reactions that have occurred in the past. Also ask what the allergic reaction actually involved. Often the patient confuses an allergy with the side effect of a drug.

Health maintenance

Determine the immunisation status (diphtheria, tetanus, pertussis (DTP), herpes simplex virus (HSV), rubella, polio, mumps, measles, influenza, *Haemophilus influenzae* and hepatitis B). Ask about past screening tests, such as Papanicolaou's (PAP) smear, mammography, chest X-rays, faecal occult blood testing, sigmoidoscopy or colonoscopy.

Menstrual and reproductive history

This information is particularly relevant for a woman with abdominal pain, a suspected endocrine disease or genitourinary symptoms. Write down the date of the last menstrual period. Ask about the age at which menstruation began, whether the periods are regular, or whether menopause has occurred. Do not forget to ask a woman in the childbearing years whether there is a possibility of pregnancy; this, for example, may preclude the use of certain investigations (e.g. involving X-rays) or drugs.

The reproductive history can be written in shorthand, as: *gravida, para, X-X-X-X*. The gravida is the total number of pregnancies (including a current one), para is the number of deliveries after 20 weeks of pregnancy, and X-X-X-X refers to the number of full-term infants, the number of pre-term infants, the number of abortions and the number of living children, respectively.

Social history (SH)

This history includes the whole economic, social, domestic and industrial situation of the patient. Ask first about the **place of birth** and **residence**. Determine the **level of education** obtained. **Ethnic background** is important in predisposing to some diseases, such as thalassaemia and sickle cell anaemia.

Occupation

Ask the patient about his or her present occupation. Sometimes finding out exactly what the patient does at work can be very important. Note particularly any work exposure to dusts, chemicals or disease; for example, mine workers may have the disease silicosis. It is also useful to find out whether the patient has a sedentary or physically active job as this will have implications for return to work after an illness. Checking on hobbies can also be informative (e.g. bird fanciers and lung disease).

Marital status, social support and living conditions

Ask who lives at home with the patient in order to ascertain the patient's marital status or other living arrangements and the home environment. Inquire whether there is anyone to help with convalescence. Find out about the health of the spouse or partner and of any children.

Social habits

This is the time when possibly awkward questions about the patient's habits should be asked.

Smoking

The patient may claim to be a non-smoker if he or she stopped smoking that morning. Therefore, you must ask whether the patient has ever smoked and, if so, how many cigarettes (or cigars or pipes) were smoked a day and for how many years. This is often recorded in packet years. A standard packet of cigarettes is considered to be 20. Twenty cigarettes a day for 20 years would therefore be 20 packet years of smoking. Cigarette smoking is a risk factor for vascular disease, chronic lung disease and several cancers, and may damage the fetus.

Alcohol

Ask whether the patient drinks alcohol. It is useful to ask first what the patient usually drinks (e.g. beer or wine) and then how many glasses a day. It can be useful at this stage to 'adjust up' the patient's estimate (e.g. 'So you drink about 10 beers a day, do you drink any spirits?'), giving the patient the chance to modify the original claim without embarrassment.

Remember the maximum safe levels of consumption recommended by the Royal College of Physicians—21 units a week for men and 14 units a week for women; 1 unit = 8 g of alcohol or just under one standard drink (one glass of wine, one glass of standard beer or one nip of spirits).

Certain questions can be helpful in making a diagnosis of alcoholism; these are referred to as the **CAGE** questions (see box). If the patient answers yes to any two of these questions, this suggests alcohol dependence is very likely, and further inquiry into the history of alcohol use from the patient and possibly the relatives becomes important.

CAGE questions

1   Have you ever felt you ought to **C**ut down on your drinking?
2   Have people **A**nnoyed you by criticising your drinking?
3   Have you ever felt bad or **G**uilty about your drinking?
4   Have you ever had a drink first thing in the morning to steady your nerves or get rid of a hangover (**E**ye opener)?

Analgesics

If the patient has not already volunteered information about the use of analgesics, ask about this. Aspirin and other non-steroidal anti-inflammatory drugs (NSAIDs), but not paracetamol (acetaminophen), can cause peptic ulcers, gastrointestinal bleeding (COX–2 selective inhibitors much less than traditional NSAIDs), asthma and renal impairment. Most NSAIDs (but not aspirin) increase the risk of myocardial infarction.

Overseas travel

If an infectious disease is a possibility, ask about recent overseas travel, destinations visited, how the patient lived when away and prophylaxis given to protect against diseases such as malaria. People who were born or have lived for long periods overseas may acquire diseases such as tuberculosis.

Sexual and drug abuse history

The patient's sexual history is relevant, particularly if there is a history of urethral discharge, dysuria (burning or pain on urination), vaginal discharge, a genital ulcer or rash, pain on intercourse or anorectal symptoms, or if the acquired immunodeficiency syndrome (AIDS) or hepatitis is suspected.

Approaching this topic is never easy for the doctor or patient. You may wish to preface these questions with a statement such as: 'I need to ask you some personal questions because they may be relevant to your current state of health.' It is not your role to make judgements about a person's life.

If a sexually transmitted disease may be the problem, a detailed sexual history will be required. Determine the last date of intercourse, number of contacts, homosexual or bisexual partners, and contacts with prostitutes. The type of sexual practice may also be important: for example, oro-anal contact may predispose to colonic infection, and peri-rectal contact to hepatitis B or C or HIV infection, while inserting objects into the rectum may cause trauma that is otherwise difficult to explain.

The use of intravenous drugs has many implications for the patient's health. If the patient uses such drugs, ask whether an attempt is made to avoid the sharing of needles. This may protect against the injection of viruses but not against bacterial infection from the use of impure substances.

Family history (FH)

Many diseases run in families. For example, ischaemic heart disease in parents who developed this at a young age is a major risk factor for ischaemic heart disease in their offspring. Various malignancies, such as breast and colon carcinoma, are more common in certain families. It is worth asking specifically about a family history of heart disease, stroke, diabetes, alcoholism or bleeding tendencies. Some diseases are directly inherited (e.g. haemophilia). Ask whether similar illnesses have occurred in other family members, but ignore long stories about suspected exotic illnesses in distant cousins.

Systems review (SR)

As well as detailed questioning about the system likely to be diseased, it is essential to ask about important symptoms and disorders in other systems, or otherwise important diseases may be missed. The extent of this review depends on the presenting problem and circumstances. An 18-year-old man needing sutures removed will clearly require less interrogation than a 75-year-old with multiple medical problems.

Ask, where relevant, about key symptoms and common disorders in each major system, but begin with some general questions as described below. Then begin the questioning for each system with a general question about any history of heart or lung trouble and so on. Decide how detailed the questioning needs to be: it is not usually necessary to ask all the listed questions.

General questions
- Have you lost or gained weight recently?
- Have there been changes in your appetite?
- Have there been changes in your pattern of sleep?
- Have you felt your mood has changed?
- Have you noticed shivering or sweating at night or had a high temperature?

Cardiovascular system
- Have you had any pain or pressure in your chest? Does this occur during exertion (angina)?
- Are you short of breath on exertion (dyspnoea)? How much exertion is necessary? How many flights of stairs can you climb before you start to become short of breath?
- Have you ever been woken at night by shortness of breath (paroxysmal nocturnal dyspnoea)?
- Can you lie flat without feeling breathless (orthopnoea)?
- Have you had swelling of your ankles (peripheral oedema), or varicose veins?
- Have you noticed your heart racing or beating irregularly?
- Do you have pain in your calves on walking (claudication)?
- Do you have cold or blue hands or feet (peripheral cyanosis)?
- Have you had rheumatic fever, a heart attack or high blood pressure?
- Also ask about specific cardiovascular risk factors:
  - Has your cholesterol level been checked recently? (If so, has it been treated or untreated?)
  - Have you been diagnosed with diabetes mellitus? (If so, for how long?)
  - Do you smoke? (If so, for how long, how many?)
  - Do you have a family history of cardiovascular disease? (If so, who and at what age?)

Respiratory system
- Are you short of breath at rest?
- Have you had any cough?
- Do you cough up anything (productive cough)?
- Have you coughed up blood (haemoptysis)?
- Do you snore loudly or fall asleep during the day unexpectedly (possible obstructive sleep apnoea)?

- Do you ever have wheezing when you are short of breath (bronchospasm)?
- Do you have night sweats?
- Have you had pneumonia or tuberculosis?
- Have you had a recent chest X-ray?

Gastrointestinal system
- Have you had a sore tongue or mouth ulcers?
- Are you troubled by indigestion? What do you mean by indigestion?
- Have you had any difficulty swallowing (dysphagia)?
- Has your appetite or weight changed? How has it changed?
- Have you had episodes of burning discomfort in the chest that rises up towards the neck (heartburn)?
- Have you been taking antacids or over-the-counter indigestion medicines?
- Have you had pain or discomfort in your belly (tummy)?
- Have you had any bloating or visible swelling of your belly?
- Has your bowel habit changed recently?
- How many bowel motions a day do you usually pass?
- Have you lost control of your bowels or had accidents (faecal incontinence)?
- Have you seen blood in your motions or on wiping (haematochezia), or vomited blood (haematemesis)?
- Have your bowel motions been black (melaena)?
- Do you take laxatives or use enemas?
- Have your eyes or skin ever been yellow (jaundice)?
- Have you noticed dark urine and pale stools?
- Have you had hepatitis, peptic ulceration, colitis or bowel cancer?
- Tell me about your diet recently.

Genitourinary system and sexual health
- Do you have burning or pain on passing urine (dysuria)?
- Is your urine stream as good as it used to be?
- Is there a delay before you start to pass urine (hesitancy)?
- Is there dribbling at the end when you pass urine?
- Do you have to get up at night to pass urine (nocturia)?
- Are you passing larger or smaller amounts of urine?
- Have you noticed leaking of urine (incontinence)?
- Has your urine colour changed? Is your urine dark?
- Have you seen blood in your urine (haematuria)?
- Have you had a urinary tract infection or kidney stones?
- Do you have any problems with your sex life?
- Have you noticed any rashes or lumps on your genitals?
- Have you had a sexually transmitted disease?
- Do you have difficulty maintaining an erection?
- Have you had a penile discharge or skin lesions?
- Have you ever felt lumps in your testes?
- Are your periods regular? At what age did you begin to menstruate (menarche)?

- Do you have excessive pain (dysmenorrhoea) or bleeding (menorrhagia) with your periods?
- Do you have bleeding after sex?
- Have you had any miscarriages?
- Have you had high blood pressure or diabetes in pregnancy?

Breasts (women)
- Have you had any bleeding or discharge from your breasts?
- Have you felt any lumps there?
- Have you had a recent mammogram or breast examination?

Haematological system
- Do you bruise easily?
- Have you had bleeding from your gums?
- Have you had fevers, or shivers and shakes (rigors)?
- Do you have difficulty stopping a small cut from bleeding?
- Have you noticed any lumps under your arms, or in your neck or groin (lymphadenopathy)?
- Have you had blood clots in your legs (venous thrombosis) or lungs (pulmonary embolism)?
- Have you had anaemia?

Musculoskeletal system
- Do you have painful or swollen joints? What joints are affected?
- Do you suffer from morning stiffness? How long does it last?
- Are your joints ever hot or red or swollen?
- Have you had muscle pains or cramps?
- Have you had a skin rash recently?
- Do you have any back or neck pain?
- Have your eyes been dry or red?
- Is your mouth often dry (Sjögren's syndrome)?
- Have you been diagnosed as having rheumatoid arthritis or gout?
- Do your fingers ever become painful and go white, then blue, then red in the cold (Raynaud's phenomenon)?
- How much do your joint problems interfere with normal activities?

Endocrine system
- Have you noticed any swelling in your neck (goitre)?
- Do your hands tremble (tremor)?
- Do you prefer hot or cold weather?
- Have you had a thyroid problem or diabetes?
- Have you noticed increased sweating?
- Have you been troubled by fatigue?
- Have you noticed any change in your appearance, hair, skin or voice?
- Have you noticed a change in hat, glove or shoe size (acromegaly)?
- Have you been unusually thirsty lately?
- Have you been passing large amounts of urine (polyuria)?

Neurological system

- Do you get headaches?
- Have you had memory problems or trouble concentrating?
- Have you had fainting episodes, fits or blackouts?
- Do you have double vision (diplopia) or other trouble seeing or hearing?
- Are you dizzy? Does the world seem to turn around (vertigo)?
- Have you had weakness, numbness or clumsiness in your arms or legs, or trouble with balance or walking?
- Have you had a stroke or serious head injury?
- Have you had difficulty sleeping?
- Do you feel sad or depressed or have problems with your nerves?
- Have you ever considered suicide?

Skin

- Have you had itching (pruritus) or a rash?
- Have you noticed moles that have changed?
- Has there been a change in your hair or nails?
- Have you had lumps or frequent infections in the skin?

Concluding the interview

Always ask the patient: 'Is anything else troubling you?' Sometimes you'll be amazed by the new information gleaned. At the end of the assessment ask the patient whether he or she has any questions, and whether there are any close relatives or friends who should be involved in the subsequent discussion about your recommendations.

Explain the next steps to the patient after making your recommendations. A clinician whose recommendations are repeatedly rejected by his or her patient has probably made a poor attempt at explaining them.

Evidence-based medicine

Evidence for the sensitivity and specificity of history taking is beginning to accumulate. High likelihood ratios for the presence of certain conditions are associated with classical symptoms. The studies indicate that more diagnoses are made from the history than from the physical examination and investigations combined.

Taking a better history (hints for success)

Listen to the patient. He is telling you the diagnosis.
Sir William Osler (1849–1919)

1. Allow the patient to tell the story in his or her own words. Establish rapport and listen with enthusiasm. Next ask specific questions to fill in the gaps. Then ask the patient whether there is *anything else* he or she would like to discuss.

2. Make sure the patient does *not* have the impression that the interview is being hurried (except in an emergency).

3. Concentrate on the history of the presenting illness. This must be documented sequentially and in the greatest detail.

4. Incorporate the relevant symptoms obtained in the systems review into the history of the presenting illness.

5. Remember that the past history, social history and family history are often highly relevant to the presenting illness.

6. Explore psychological issues where they may be relevant.

7. Don't accept one-line answers and don't be content with facts that seem contradictory or chronologically obscure; trust, but verify always.

8. Use systematic questions about potential risk factors for various diseases to assist in establishing the diagnosis (e.g. smoking and coronary artery disease).

9. Remember that constant practice is needed to become a proficient history taker.

10. A good interview has therapeutic value.

chapter 2

Advanced history taking

Whatever I see or hear, professionally or privately, which ought not to be divulged, I will keep secret and tell no one.

Hippocratic oath

Certain aspects of history taking go beyond routine questioning about symptoms. This part of the art has to be learned by taking lots of histories; practice is absolutely essential. With time you will gain confidence in dealing with patients whose psychiatric, cultural or medical situation makes standard questioning difficult or impossible.

Personal history taking

Most illnesses are stressful and can induce feelings of anxiety or depression. On the other hand, patients with primary psychiatric illnesses often present with physical not psychological symptoms. The **brain–body interaction is bidirectional**, and you need to understand this as you obtain the patient's story.

The patient may be reluctant or initially unable to discuss sensitive problems with a stranger. Gaining the patient's confidence is critical. Although this type of history taking can be difficult, it can also be the most satisfying of all interviews, since interviewing can be directly therapeutic for the patient.

A **sympathetic, unhurried approach** using **open-ended questions** will provide much information that can then be systematically recorded after the interview. It is important that you maintain an objective demeanour, particularly when asking about delicate subjects, such as sexual problems, grief reactions or abuse.

The formal **psychiatric interview** differs from general medical history taking. It often takes considerable time for patients to develop rapport with, and confidence in, the clinician. There are certain standard questions that may give valuable insights into the patient's state of mind (see below). It may be important to obtain much more detailed information about each of these problems, depending on the clinical circumstances.

Sympathetic confrontation can be helpful in some situations. For example, if the patient appears sad, angry or frightened, referring to this in a tactful way may lead the patient to volunteer appropriate information. If an emotional response is obtained, use emotional-handling skills (**NURS**) to deal with this during the interview (see box).

NURS

- *Name* the emotion.
- Show *Understanding*.
- Deal with the issue with *Respect*.
- Show *Support*.
  (For example: 'It makes sense you were angry after your husband left you. This must have been very difficult to deal with. Can I be of any help to you now?')

Personal history: useful questions to ask

- Where do you live (e.g. a house, flat or hostel)?
- Tell me about your current work and where you have worked in the past.
- Do you get on well with people at home?
- Do you get on well with people at work?
- Do you have any financial problems?
- Are you married or have you been married?
- Could you tell me about your close relationships?
- Would you describe your marriage (or living arrangements) as happy?
- Have you been hit, kicked or physically hurt by someone (physical abuse)?
- Have you been forced to have sex (sexual abuse)?
- Would you say you have a large number of friends?
- Are you religious?
- Do you feel you are too fat or too thin?
- Has anyone in the family had problems with psychiatric illness?
- Have you ever had a nervous breakdown?
- Have you ever had any psychiatric problem?

Symptoms of depression: useful questions to ask

- Have you been feeling sad, down or blue?
- Have you felt depressed or lost interest in things daily for two or more weeks in the past?
- Have you ever felt like taking your own life?
- Have you had early morning wakening?
- Has your appetite been poor recently?
- Have you lost weight recently?

- How do you feel about the future?
- Have you had trouble concentrating on things?
- Have you had guilty thoughts?
- Have you lost interest in things you usually enjoy?

Symptoms of anxiety: useful questions to ask

- Do you worry excessively about things?
- Do you have trouble relaxing?
- Do you have problems getting to sleep at night?
- Do you feel uncomfortable in crowded places?
- Do you worry excessively about minor things?
- Do you feel suddenly frightened or anxious or panicky for no reason in situations in which most people would not be afraid?
- Do you find you have to do things repetitively, such as washing your hands multiple times?
- Do you have any rituals (such as checking things) that you feel you have to do, even though you know it may be silly?
- Do you have recurrent thoughts that you have trouble controlling?

Cultural history taking

Attitudes to illness and disease vary in different cultures. Problems considered shameful by the patient may be very difficult for him or her to discuss. In some cultures (and increasingly in Australia) women may object to being, or it may not be acceptable for women to be, questioned or examined by male doctors or students. Male students may need to be accompanied by a **female chaperone** when interviewing a sensitive female patient and should have a female chaperone when undertaking the patient's physical examination. It is most important that cultural sensitivities on either side do not prevent a thorough medical assessment.

Aboriginal patients may have a large extended family. These relatives may be able to provide invaluable support to the patient, but the medical or social problems may interfere with the patient's ability to manage his or her own health. Commitments to family members may make it difficult for a patient to attend medical appointments or travel for specialist treatment. Detailed questioning about family contacts and responsibilities may help with the planning of the patient's treatment.

For patients who speak little English, use of an official medical interpreter is appropriate. The need for an interpreter makes history taking more time-consuming and difficult. It is better to avoid using a patient's relative as an interpreter if possible, to reduce bias. Professional medical translators are trained not to reinterpret the patient's history and have a good knowledge of medical terms. Learn to make eye contact with the patient rather than the interpreter during the interview, otherwise the patient may feel left out of the discussion. Questions should be directed as if going straight to the patient: 'Have you had any problems with shortness of breath?' rather than 'Has he had any breathlessness?'

It is alarmingly common for relatives who accompany patients to interrupt and contradict the patient's version of events. The interposition of a relative between the clinician and the patient always makes the history taking less direct and the patient's symptoms more subject to 'filtering' or interpretation before the information reaches the clinician. Try tactfully to direct the relative to allow the patient to answer in his or her own words.

All these issues require an especially sensitive approach. As a clinician you need to be impartial and objective. You may need to discuss specific issues with members of the medical faculty and find out what the university and hospital policies are on such matters.

Functional history taking: activities and instrumental activities of daily living

Elderly patients and patients with chronic disabling illnesses need to have their ability to manage normal living assessed (**activities of daily living, ADLs**). As part of the review of such a patient's symptoms, ask basic screening questions that include the patient's ability to bathe, walk, use the toilet, and eat and dress. Also ask questions about the **instrumental activities of daily living (IADLs)**, such as shopping, cooking and cleaning, using transport, and managing money and medications. This assessment extends beyond medical diagnosis so that the clinician can accurately judge the patient's social and domestic circumstances.

Related questions about the patient's domestic arrangements will be important if the ADLs are limited. The number of steps in the house, the provision of railings in the bathroom and the accessibility of cupboards may all be important. Ask about access to transport for shopping and medical treatment and the availability of help for housework and cooking. Find out who else lives with the patient and how those people seem to be coping with the patient's illness. Obviously the amount of detail required depends on the severity and chronicity of the patient's illness.

The 'difficult' patient

Most clinical encounters are a cooperative effort on the part of the patient and clinician. The patient wants help to find out what is wrong and to get better. However, interviews do not always run smoothly. **Resentment** may occur on both sides if the patient seems not to be taking the doctor's advice seriously, or will not cooperate with attempts at history taking or examination. Unless there is a serious psychiatric or neurological problem that impairs the patient's judgement, this remains the patient's prerogative.

Always remember that as a clinician you have a duty to **give advice and explanation**, not to dictate. Indeed, it is arrogant to assume that your advice is always right. Patients who seem sceptical about what they are being advised must always be given the chance to think things over and to seek other opinions. This approach, however, must not be used as an excuse for not providing a proper, sympathetic and thorough explanation of the

2

problem and the consequences of ignoring medical advice—to the extent that the patient will allow.

Patients who are **aggressive** and uncooperative may have a medical reason for their behaviour. The possibilities to be considered include alcohol or drug withdrawal, an intracranial lesion such as a tumour or subdural haematoma, or a psychiatric disease such as paranoid schizophrenia. In other cases, resentment at the occurrence of illness may be the problem.

Some patients may seem difficult because they are *too* **cooperative**. The patient concerned about his blood pressure may have brought printouts of his own blood pressure measurements at half-hour intervals for several weeks. It is important to show restrained interest in these recordings without encouraging excessive enthusiasm. Other patients may bring with them information about their symptoms or a diagnosis obtained from the internet. It is important to remember, and perhaps to point out, that information obtained in this way may not have been subjected to any form of peer review. People with chronic illnesses, on the other hand, may know more about their conditions than their clinician.

Sometimes the interests of the patient and the doctor are not the same. This is especially so in cases where there is the possibility of compensation for an illness or injury. Such patients may, consciously or unconsciously, attempt to **manipulate the encounter**. This is a very difficult problem and can be approached only with rigorous application of clinical methods.

Occasionally, attempted manipulation takes the form of flattery or inappropriate personal interest directed at the clinician. This should be dealt with by maintaining careful professional detachment. The clinician and the patient must be conscious that their meeting is strictly professional and not social.

History taking for the maintenance of good health

The first interview with a patient is an opportunity to make an assessment of the known risk factors for a number of important medical conditions (see box below). Even when a patient has come about an unconnected problem, there is often the opportunity for a quick review of these factors. Constant matter-of-fact reminders about these issues can make a great deal of difference to the way people protect themselves from ill-health.

Most people have some understanding of the dangers associated with smoking, excessive alcohol consumption and obesity. People have more varied views on what constitutes a healthy diet and exercise regimen, and many are ignorant of what constitutes risky sexual activity. Part of the thorough assessment of a patient includes obtaining and conveying some idea of what measures may help the patient to maintain good health. This includes a comprehensive approach to the combination of risk factors for various diseases, which are much more important than individual risk factors. For example, advising a patient about his or her risk of premature cardiovascular disease will involve knowing about the patient's family history, smoking history, previous and current blood pressure, current and historical cholesterol levels, dietary history, assessment for diabetes and level of exercise undertaken.

Ask whether the patient has undergone a screening test for colon cancer. A strong family history of carcinoma of the colon may be an indication for screening colonoscopy at an age earlier than 50 years. Women should be asked about their family history of certain malignancies such as carcinoma of the breast or ovary, and about previous screening tests for these conditions.

The patient's vaccination record should also be reviewed regularly and brought up to date when indicated.

Useful routine questions to help patients to maintain good health
Ask patients about the following:
- Smoking habits and cholesterol level
- Diet and consumption of alcohol
- Level of exercise
- Current weight, and any recent change in weight
- Practices related to sexual health
- Vaccinations (for adults over 18 years of age; also see www.cdc.gov/vaccines/recs/schedules/adult-schedule.htm):
  - *Haemophilus influenzae* type b
  - hepatitis A and B
  - human papilloma virus (females ≤ 26 years only)
  - influenza (annually, if at increased risk)
  - measles, mumps, rubella
  - meningococcal
  - pneumococcal
  - tetanus, diphtheria, pertussis (every 10 years)
  - varicella zoster (60 years and older)
- Screening for breast cancer and ovarian cancer (family history, or age 50 years plus)
- Screening for colon cancer (age 50 years plus, or family history of colon cancer or personal history of inflammatory bowel disease)
- Family history of other inherited diseases (may be an indication for screening tests, e.g. hypertrophic cardiomyopathy)
- Family history of sudden death

History taking OSCE: hints panel

The objective structured clinical examination (OSCE) is an evaluation tool used to assess some or all of the following: history taking skills, clinical examination skills, communication skills with patients and families, data interpretation, ability to document information, ability to infer the differential diagnosis and technical skills. It consists of numerous stations, and students move from station to station on the same timetable, spending 10–15 minutes at each one. Each station is scored separately and scores are combined to determine the pass level.

A number of history taking skills can be tested. A real patient or an actor may be available to answer questions and enable the examiner to test your interviewing technique and knowledge. An approach to some of these questions is summarised here as an example.

Begin all interviews by introducing yourself. In most cases the first question should probably be 'May I ask you some questions?' or 'May I have a look at you?'

1 **Question this patient about her risk factors for cardiovascular disease.**

(a) Ask her the following:
   (i)   What is your date of birth?
   (ii) Do you have a previous history of cardiovascular disease or high blood pressure?
   (iii) What is your cholesterol level? (Has it been treated or untreated?)
   (iv) Do you have diabetes? (If so, for how long?)
   (v)   Do you smoke? (If so, for how long? How many?)
   (vi) Do you have a family history of cardiovascular disease? (If so, who was affected and at what age?)

(b) Synthesise and present your findings.

2 **This man is short of breath. Take a history from him about this.**

(a) Ask him the following:
   (i)   When are you short of breath (on exertion; lying flat—orthopnoea or paroxysmal nocturnal dyspnoea)?
   (ii) How bad is it? (grade I–IV)
   (iii) How long does it last? Is it getting worse? Do you have any associated symptoms (e.g. wheeze, chest tightness)?
   (iv) Do you have cough? Fever? Pleuritic chest pain?
   (v)   Have you had previous heart or lung disease?
   (vi) Do you smoke? (If so, for how long? How many?)

(b) Synthesise and present your findings.

3 **This man has chronic rheumatoid arthritis. Assess his social situation.**

(a) Ask him the following:
   (i)   How long have you been affected?
   (ii)   Which joints are affected?
   (iii) Can you bathe yourself, go to toilet, dress yourself, cut food, eat (ADLs)?
   (iv)   How do you manage shopping, cooking, cleaning, transport and driving, managing medications and finances (IADLs)?
   (v)   Do you work?
   (vi)   Who lives at home?
   (vii) What support do you get?
   (viii) What is the layout of your house (are there rails, steps etc)?

(b) Synthesise and present your findings.

4 **This woman has been having problems with depression. Would you take a history from her?**

(a) Ask her the following:
   (i)   Have you been feeling sad? How long?
   (ii) Have you felt depressed or lost interest in things daily for two or more weeks in the past?

  (iii) Is there any particular precipitating problem?
  (iv) Do you have early morning wakening?
  (v)   Do you suffer from loss of appetite or weight?
  (vi) What are your thoughts about the future?
  (vii) Are you able to concentrate?
  (viii)Do you have guilty thoughts?
  (ix) Have you experienced loss of interest in things you usually enjoy?
  (x)   Have you ever thought of killing yourself? Have you thought what
        you might do?
  (xi) What treatment have you had?
  (xii) Do you have a history of major medical problems like cancer?
(b) Synthesise and present your findings.

Taking a better history hints for success

1 Ask open questions to start with (and resist the urge to interrupt), but finish with specific questions to narrow the differential diagnosis.
2 Do not hurry (or at least do not appear to be in a hurry, even if you have only limited time).
3 Ask the patient 'What else?' after he or she has finished speaking, to ensure that all problems have been identified. Repeat the 'What else?' question as often as required.
4 Keep comfortable eye contact and an open posture.
5 Use the head nod appropriately, and use silences to encourage the patient to express himself or herself.
6 When there are breaks in the narrative, provide a summary for the patient, by briefly restating the facts or feelings identified, to maximise accuracy and demonstrate active listening.
7 Clarify the list of chief or presenting complaints with the patient, rather than assuming that you know them.
8 If you are confused about the chronology of events or other issues, admit it and ask the patient to clarify.
9 Make sure the patient's story is internally consistent and, if not, ask more questions to verify the facts.
10 If emotions are uncovered, *name* the patient's emotion and indicate that you *understand* (e.g. 'you seem sad'), show *respect* and express your *support* (e.g. 'it's understandable that you would feel upset').
11 Ask about any other concerns the patient may have and address specific fears.
12 Express your support and willingness to cooperate with the patient to help solve the problems together.

Beginning the examination

Observe, record, tabulate, communicate: use your five senses.
Sir William Osler (1849–1919)

When you hear hoof beats, think of horses not zebras.
The Zebra Rule

It is thrilling to search for objective evidence of disease (physical signs). To do this well you need to develop your own systematic technique. As you find abnormalities, you will need to decide the likely diagnostic possibilities so that you can search for other clues to support or refute your differential diagnosis. Remember, common things are common so, considering the patient's age and sex, think about the most frequent possibilities first when formulating your differential (hence the Zebra Rule above).

Equipment

A sense of excitement usually accompanies the acquisition of examination tools by the new medical student, but resist purchasing exotic and expensive equipment. This is not only unnecessary, but it also may be unwise to present on the first day with a gold-plated stethoscope clearly superior to that of the teaching staff; it leaves very little excuse for not being able to hear soft murmurs.

Most students equip themselves with a number of frequently used items. The most glamorous and indeed most useful (except for the only really vital tool, a pen) is the stethoscope. Many types are available and most work well. It is said that it is what is between the ear-pieces of the stethoscope that really matters. There is some advantage in having a separate tube for each ear. These may be bound in a single outer tube or separated, but they should not bounce together and make distracting noises. The stethoscope needs to be robust and easily squashed into different-sized pockets.

It must also be comfortable when worn in the current fashionable position (e.g. slung around the neck). Some newer models do not have a separate bell and diaphragm.

Most other equipment can be obtained on the wards but it is worth acquiring a small pocket ophthalmoscope, a torch and a short patellar hammer. More senior students can usually give advice about the most reliable and inexpensive models available.

General appearance

Before the specific examination of the regions or medical systems of the body begins, a general inspection must be made. Make a conscious effort and take the time to consider the patient's appearance, including the **face** (see Table 3.1), **hands** (see Table 3.2) and **body**. Certain facies and body habituses are diagnostic or nearly so. Important relevant signs may be missed unless this is done (seeing the wood rather than the trees). For example, the patient with loss of weight may not be identified as having thyrotoxicosis (see Ch 9) unless the eye signs (e.g. thyroid stare) are noticed.

Table 3.1 Some important diagnostic facies	
Acromegalic • Prominent chin • Supra-orbital ridges	
Cushingoid • Plethoric and fat	
Down syndrome • Epicanthic folds • Large tongue	

Table 3.1 **Some important diagnostic facies** *continued*

Hippocratic (advanced peritonitis)
- Eyes are sunken
- Temples collapsed
- Nose is pinched with crusts on the lips
- Forehead is clammy

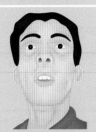

Marfanoid
- Thin, high arched palate

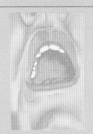

Mitral
- Malar flush (bluish discolouration over the cheeks)

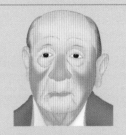

Myopathic (dystrophia myotonica)
- Frontal balding
- Triangular, wasted masseters
- Thick spectacles or intra-ocular lens implantation

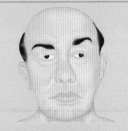

Myxoedematous
- Puffy
- Lacking in expression
- Skin thickening
- Thinning hair
- Loss of outer one-third of eyebrows

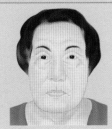

continued

Table 3.1 Some important diagnostic facies *continued*

Pagetic • Large cranium	
Parkinsonian • Expressionless • Infrequent blinking	
Thyrotoxic • Thyroid stare • Lid retraction • Exophthalmos	
Virile facies • Acne • Facial hair in women	

Table 3.2 Nail signs in systemic disease

Nail sign	Some causes
Blue nails	Cyanosis, Wilson's disease, ochronosis
Red nails	Polycythaemia (reddish-blue), carbon monoxide poisoning (cherry red)
Clubbing	Lung cancer, chronic pulmonary suppuration, infective endocarditis, cyanotic congenital heart disease
Splinter haemorrhages	Infective endocarditis, vasculitis

Table 3.2 **Nail signs in systemic disease** *continued*	
Koilonychia (spoon-shaped nails)	Iron deficiency
Pale nail bed	Anaemia
Onycholysis (separation of nail from nail bed)	Thyrotoxicosis, psoriasis
Leuconychia (white nails)	Hypoalbuminaemia
Nail fold erythema	Systemic lupus erythematosus and telangiectasia

First impressions

Is the patient relatively well or very ill? Specific abnormalities will sometimes be recognised. Look particularly for **jaundice** (yellow discolouration of the skin and sclerae), **cyanosis** (blue discolouration of the skin), **pallor** (suggesting anaemia) or one of the **diagnostic facies** (see Table 3.1).

Vital signs

These are indicators of the function of essential parts of the body. They should be assessed in all patients at the time of the initial examination and then as often as necessary.

1. Examine the **radial pulse** (see Fig 3.1). It is usually palpable just medial to the distal radius with the pulps of the forefinger and middle finger of the examining hand. Estimate or count the rate and note the rhythm (see p. 55).

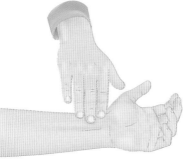

Figure 3.1 Taking the radial pulse

2. Measure the **blood pressure** (see Fig 3.2). The normal blood pressure **cuff width** is 12.5 cm. This is suitable for a normal-sized adult upper arm. However, in obese patients with large arms, this cuff will overestimate the blood pressure and therefore a large cuff must be used. A range of smaller sizes is available for children.

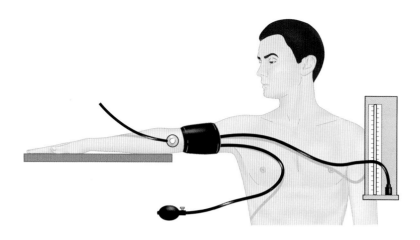

Phase	Korotkoff sounds	
		120 mmHg systotic
1	A thud	
		110 mmHg
2	A blowing noise	
		100 mmHg
3	A softer thud	
		90 mmHg diastolic (1st)
4	A disappearing blowing noise	
		80 mmHg diastolic (2nd)
5	Nothing	

Figure 3.2 Taking the blood pressure

The cuff is wrapped around the **upper arm** (which should be **supported at the level of the heart**) and the **bladder centred over the brachial artery**. This is found in the antecubital fossa immediately medial to the biceps tendon.

For an approximate estimation of the systolic blood pressure, the cuff is fully inflated and then deflated slowly (2 mmHg per second) until the radial pulse returns (**palpation method**). Then, for a more accurate estimation of the blood pressure, this manoeuvre is repeated with the stethoscope placed over the brachial artery (**auscultation method**). You must master both methods.

Five sounds will be heard as the cuff is slowly released (see Fig 3.2). These are called the **Korotkoff sounds**. The pressure at which a sound is first heard over the artery is the systolic blood pressure (Korotkoff I [K I]). As deflation of the cuff continues the sound increases in intensity (K II), then decreases (K III), becomes muffled (K IV) and then disappears (K V). Disappearance (K V) is normally taken to indicate the level of the diastolic pressure. A normal *auscultatory gap* may sometimes occur (the sounds disappear just below systolic pressure but reappear above diastolic).

The systolic blood pressure may normally vary between the arms by up to 10 mmHg; in the **legs**, where it can be taken with a special large cuff placed over the thigh (the popliteal artery is used instead of the brachial), the blood pressure is normally higher than in the arms (this is not routine). However, if coarctation of the aorta or subclavian artery stenosis is suspected, these readings may be performed.

Optimal blood pressure: < 120 mmHg systolic; < 80 mmHg diastolic.
High normal blood pressure: 130–139 mmHg systolic; and/or 85–89 mmHg diastolic.
Mild hypertension (grade 1): 140–159 mmHg systolic; and/or 90–99 mmHg diastolic.
Moderate hypertension (grade 2): 160–179 mmHg systolic; and/or 100–109 mmHg diastolic.
Severe hypertension (grade 3): ≥ 180 mmHg systolic; and /or ≥ 110 mmHg diastolic.

Blood pressure measured at home by the patient or with a 24-hour monitor will confirm office readings that may be artificially high (**white-coat hypertension**, so-called because doctors all used to wear white coats).

During inspiration, the systolic and diastolic blood pressures normally decrease. When this normal reduction in blood pressure with inspiration is exaggerated, it is termed **pulsus paradoxus**. A fall of more than 10 mmHg in arterial pulse pressure on inspiration is abnormal and may occur with constrictive pericarditis, pericardial effusion or severe asthma. To measure pulsus paradoxus, lower the cuff slowly and note when the K I sound is occurring intermittently (expiration), then lower the cuff further until K I is audible with every beat; the difference equals the pulsus paradoxus.

3. Take the **temperature**. A mercury thermometer is shaken and then placed under the tongue, in the axilla or sometimes in the rectum for 2 minutes and then read. Electronic thermometers, which are often used to take the temperature in the ear and beep in a helpful way when ready, have replaced mercury ones in many hospitals. The normal temperature in the mouth and ear is 37 °C and is about 1 °C less in the axilla and about 1 °C more if taken in the rectum.

4. Count the **respiratory rate**. The normal rate is between 16 and 25 breaths per minute. An increased rate may be due to lung disease of almost any type, cardiac failure or metabolic disturbances such as acidosis, or to psychological conditions such as anxiety.

Weight and body habitus

Look specifically for **obesity**, **wasting** (loss of muscle mass), an unusual **facial** appearance (see Table 3.1) or an **abnormal body shape** (e.g. the tall thin appearance with long fingers that occurs in Marfan's syndrome).

1. **Weigh** the patient. For children the height should also be measured and a weight–height chart consulted to determine the child's growth percentile. For adults whose weight appears abnormal, the **body mass index (BMI)** should be calculated. The formula is weight/height squared (kg/m^2). A BMI between 18.5 and 25 is normal, while $\geq$ 30 indicates obesity and < 18.5 indicates underweight.
2. Inspect for **limb deformity** or missing limbs (these are not always obvious if the patient is huddled under the bed clothes). If the patient walks into the examining room, the opportunity to examine the gait should not be lost; the full testing of gait is described in Chapter 7.
3. Assess the state of **hydration**. Severe dehydration is associated with sunken orbits, dry mucous membranes (e.g. tongue), reduced skin elasticity (turgor—an area of skin when pulled away from the body hangs in a wrinkled state for some seconds before falling back) and hypotension (low blood pressure).
4. Look for **pallor**, which may indicate anaemia, and for cyanosis (see p. 53).

The hands and nails

Examination of a system of the body often begins with inspection of the hands and nails. For example, the patient with suspected chronic liver disease may have **liver nails** (white nail beds with a rim of pink at the top) and **palmar erythema** (red palms). Nail and finger changes may also occur in cardiac and respiratory diseases, endocrine diseases (e.g. acromegaly), arthritis, neurological disease and anaemia (see Figs 3.3 and 3.4).

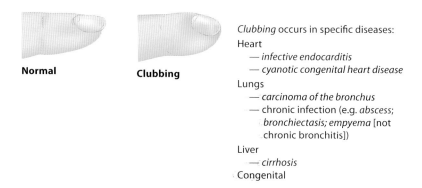

Normal   **Clubbing**

Clubbing occurs in specific diseases:
Heart
    — *infective endocarditis*
    — *cyanotic congenital heart disease*
Lungs
    — *carcinoma of the bronchus*
    — chronic infection (e.g. *abscess; bronchiectasis; empyema* [not chronic bronchitis])
Liver
    — *cirrhosis*
Congenital

Figure 3.3 Nail changes

Koilonychia

Koilonychia can occur in iron-deficiency anaemia

Splinter haemorrhages

Splinter haemorrhages occur in *infective endocarditis* but are more common in people doing manual labour

Pitting

Pitting occurs in *psoriasis* and *psoriatic arthritis*

Figure 3.3 Nail changes *continued*

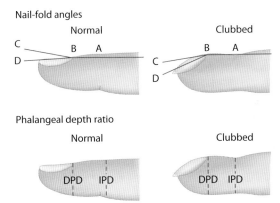

DPD = distal phalangeal depth
IPD = interphalangeal depth

Figure 3.4 Phalangeal depth ratio

How to examine a lump

Lumps may be present anywhere on the surface of the body. They are usually readily examined and you must have an approach that helps work out the cause.

1. First, look at and feel the lump to work out its **anatomical site** on the body and **its size**, **shape** and **consistency** (soft or hard). Note whether it is **tender** or not.

2. Next, work out in **what tissue layer** the lump is situated. If it is in the **skin** (e.g. sebaceous cyst, epidermoid cyst, papilloma), it should move when the skin is moved, but if it is in the **subcutaneous tissue** (e.g. neurofibroma, lipoma), the skin can be moved over the lump. If it is in the **muscle** or **tendon** (e.g. tumour), then contraction of the muscle or tendon will limit the lump's mobility, and mobility is greater in the transverse than the longitudinal axis. If it is in a **nerve**, pressing on the lump may result in pins and needles (paraesthesiae) being felt in the distribution of the nerve, and the lump cannot be moved in the longitudinal axis but can be moved in the transverse axis. If it is in **bone**, the lump will be immobile.

3. Find out whether the lump is **fluctuant** (i.e. contains fluid; see Fig. 3.5). Place two forefingers (the 'watching' fingers) halfway between the centre and periphery of the lump. The forefinger from the other hand (the 'displacing' finger) is placed diagonally opposite at an equal distance from the centre of the lump. Press with the displacing finger and keep the watching fingers still. If the lump contains fluid, the watching fingers will be displaced in **both** axes of the lump (i.e. fluctuation is present). Place a small torch behind the lump to determine whether it can be **transilluminated** (if there is fluid, light will shine through the lump).

Watching fingers

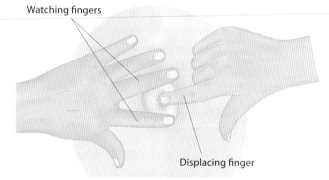

Displacing finger

Figure 3.5 Testing a lump for fluctuation

4. Note any **associated signs of inflammation** (i.e. redness, swelling, heat and tenderness).

5. Look for **similar lumps elsewhere** (e.g. multiple subcutaneous swellings from neurofibromas or lipomas). If an inflammatory or neoplastic lump is suspected, remember always to examine the regional **lymphatic field** and the other lymph node groups, as explained in Chapter 6.

Always remember to describe a lump:

- *Site*
- *Size*
- *Shape*
- *Consistency*
- *Colour*
- *Contour*
- *Tenderness*
- *Tethering*
- *Temperature*

3

Preparing the patient for examination

Try to ensure that the patient is comfortable and positioned so as to assist the examination. At each stage the patient should be informed about what is going to happen.

The patient must be undressed so that the parts to be examined are accessible. Modesty requires that a woman's breasts be covered temporarily with a gown or sheet while other parts of the body are being examined. Men and women should both have the groin covered, for example, during the examination of the legs. However, important physical signs will be missed in some patients if excessive attention is paid to modesty. The position of the patient in bed or elsewhere should depend on what is to be examined. For example, a patient's abdomen is best examined if he or she lies completely flat so that the abdominal muscles are relaxed. Traditionally, the doctor examines from the right side of the bed.

Every effort should be made to ensure that the examination is not uncomfortable or embarrassing for the patient. The curtains should be drawn around the bed and members of the clinician's entourage should be introduced. Attempt to warm your examining hands and stethoscope before they are applied to the patient's skin. Always wash your hands before and after touching a patient to protect the patient and you.

Beginning the examination OSCE: hints panel

This OSCE may involve important spot diagnoses or demonstration of important examination techniques. The examiner will usually give a very specific instruction about what is to be done. It is important to listen carefully to any introduction given about the patient. These introductions (often a brief history) are meant to help with the diagnosis.

Always perform exactly the examination requested, but begin by introducing yourself and asking the patient's permission to perform the examination. Then stand back and make a brief inspection of the patient. Some diagnoses are more obvious from a distance, and important clues such as an intravenous cannula containing antibiotics or anticoagulant may otherwise be missed.

1   **Take this patient's blood pressure (see p. 27).**

   (a) Make sure you take the blood pressure by palpation and then auscultation using the proper technique.

   (b) Check for a postural blood pressure drop (lying and sitting).

   (c) If the blood pressure is elevated, look for secondary causes of hypertension (e.g. palpate for radiofemoral delay in coarctation of the aorta, listen for a renal bruit).

   (d) Ask to look for complications of hypertension (e.g. fundoscopy changes of malignant hypertension; p. 147).

   (e) Synthesise and present your findings.

2 Examine this patient's fingernails. He is a smoker who has had recent lung problems.

This introduction suggests that the abnormality may be clubbing, possibly due to carcinoma of the lung.

(a) Stand back to look for dyspnoea.

(b) Inspect the nails (Table 3.2) from the side. Look for loss of the hyponychial angle.

(c) Note cyanosis.

(d) Look for tar staining.

(e) Examine the respiratory system (p. 67).

(f) Synthesise and present your findings.

chapter 4

The heart and cardiovascular system

Heart: The muscle which by its contraction and dilation propels the blood through the course of circulation.

S Johnson, *A Dictionary Of The English Language* **(1755)**

This chapter presents an introduction to history taking and examination of the cardiovascular system. The examination of the heart itself is described first, but it is usual to begin the examination with an assessment of the peripheral signs of cardiovascular disease, as set out below.

The cardiovascular system assessment sequence

1 Presenting symptoms, e.g. chest pain, dyspnoea, palpitations, peripheral oedema
2 Detailed questions about presenting symptoms (SOCRATES, p. 4)
3 Questions about previous cardiac problems and cardiac risk factors
4 Examination for peripheral signs of cardiovascular disease, including the pulses and blood pressure
5 Examination of the neck (carotid pulse and jugular venous pressure)
6 Examination of the praecordium including apex beat, heart sounds and murmurs
7 Examination of the lung fields for signs of cardiac failure
8 Provisional and differential diagnosis

The cardiac history

Presenting symptoms (see Table 4.1)

Chest pain

The cause of chest pain (see Table 4.2) is likely to be clearer when questions about the quality, duration, location, precipitating and aggravating factors, means of relief and accompanying symptoms have been answered. These are the same questions used to assess pain anywhere in the body.

Table 4.1 The cardiovascular history

Major symptoms
Chest pain, tightness, discomfort or heaviness
Dyspnoea: exertional (note degree of exercise necessary), orthopnoea, paroxysmal nocturnal dyspnoea
Ankle swelling
Palpitations
Syncope and dizziness
Intermittent claudication
Fatigue

Past history
Rheumatic fever, chorea, recent (past three months) dental work, thyroid disease
Prior medical examination revealing heart disease (e.g. military, school, insurance)
Drugs

Social history
Smoking habits and alcohol use

Family history
Myocardial infarcts, cardiomyopathy, congenital heart disease, mitral valve prolapse, Marfan's syndrome

Coronary artery disease risk factors
Previous coronary or vascular disease
Hyperlipidaemia
Hypertension
Smoking
Family history of coronary artery disease
Diabetes mellitus
Obesity and physical inactivity
Male sex and advanced age
Erectile dysfunction

Typical ischaemic chest pain is due to inadequate blood supply to the myocardium. It is often described as a central or retrosternal (behind the sternum) discomfort rather than a pain. There is frequently a tight or heavy sensation, which may radiate to the left arm or to the jaw. It tends to occur on exertion and may be predictable at certain levels of activity. Relief is usually rapid with rest or sublingual (under the tongue) nitrate drugs. Prolonged ischaemic-type pain or discomfort that comes on at rest is more suggestive of myocardial infarction than angina. The pain of infarction is more likely to be associated with sweating than that of angina.

Unless a careful history is taken, and the association with exertion is noted, the clinician and the patient may incorrectly assume that lower chest discomfort is due to heartburn (acid reflux) rather than to angina. Pain worse on respiration suggests pulmonary disease, whereas pain worse with movement of the upper limbs suggests musculoskeletal-type pain. Consult Table 4.2 for other causes of chest pain.

Table 4.2 Causes of chest pain and typical features	
Cardiac pain	Angina **(exertional)**, myocardial ischaemia or infarction **(persistent)**
Vascular pain	Aortic dissection **(very sudden onset, radiates to the back)**
Pleuropericardial pain	Pericarditis **(pleuritic pain, worse when patient lies down)** Infective pleurisy **(pleuritic pain, p. 65)** Pneumothorax **(sudden onset, sharp, associated with dyspnoea)** Pneumonia **(often pleuritic, associated with fever and dyspnoea)** Autoimmune disease **(pleuritic)** Mesothelioma **(severe and constant)** Metastatic tumour **(severe and constant, localised)**
Chest wall pain	Persistent cough **(worse with movement, chest wall tender)** Muscular strains **(worse with movement, chest wall tender)** Intercostal myositis **(worse with movement, chest wall tender)** Thoracic herpes zoster **(severe, follows nerve root distribution, precedes rash)** Coxsackie B virus infection **(pleuritic)** Thoracic nerve compression or infiltration **(follows nerve root distribution)** Rib fracture **(history of trauma, localised tenderness)** Rib tumour, primary or metastatic **(constant, severe, localised)** Tietze's syndrome **(costal cartilage tender)**
Gastrointestinal pain	Gastro-oesophageal reflux **(not related to exertion, burning, rises up towards the neck, may be worse when patient lies down—p. 80)** Diffuse oesophageal spasm **(rare, not exertional)**
Airway pain	Tracheitis **(pain in throat, breathing painful)** Inhaled foreign body **(stridor)**
Other causes	Panic attacks **(often preceded by anxiety, associated with breathlessness)**

Dyspnoea

Shortness of breath may be due to cardiac disease. In this case it is often associated with **orthopnoea** (breathlessness that is worse when the patient lies flat) and **paroxysmal nocturnal dyspnoea** (PND, breathlessness that wakes the patient from sleep—typically the patient gets up and walks to the window to breathe in fresh air, and it takes several minutes for relief to occur). This occurs because of a sudden failure of left ventricular output, causing transudation of fluid into the lung tissues.

Valvular heart disease and angina can also cause breathlessness. In that case, patients usually describe symptoms that are predictable with exertion but do not have orthopnoea unless heart failure has supervened. When it is due to angina, dyspnoea is often associated with a feeling of chest tightness.

Cardiac dyspnoea can be difficult to distinguish from that due to other causes, such as lung disease. It is important to find out whether the patient has a history of diseases that can cause cardiac failure (e.g. previous myocardial infarction, hypertension or valvular heart disease). Dyspnoea due to lung disease may be associated with wheezing and orthopnoea is absent.

Ankle swelling

Peripheral oedema may be a symptom (and sign) of cardiac failure, but there are other more common causes of ankle swelling (e.g. varicose veins, vasodilating drugs).

Palpitations

This is usually taken to mean an unexpected awareness of the heartbeat. Try to find out precisely what it is the patient is aware of. Ask about the perceived heart rate, the suddenness of onset and offset, and the regularity or irregularity of the heartbeat. It may help to get the patient to tap out the rhythm of the heartbeat with a finger.

Syncope and dizziness

Syncope is a **transient loss of consciousness** resulting from cerebral anoxia. It is necessary to establish whether the patient actually loses consciousness, and also under what circumstances the syncope occurs (e.g. postural syncope occurs on standing, micturition syncope occurs when the patient is passing urine, tussive syncope occurs with coughing and vasovagal syncope occurs with sudden emotional stress). The differential diagnosis includes **epilepsy**, where there may be associated tonic and clonic jerks (rhythmical contraction and relaxation of muscle groups). Aortic stenosis (p. 51) or hypertrophic cardiomyopathy (p. 52) may be associated with syncope that occurs on exertion, probably related to inappropriate vasodilatation and hypotension from stimulation of ventricular mechanoreceptors.

Dizziness that occurs even when the patient is lying down or that is made worse by movements of the head is more likely to be of neurological or middle ear origin (p. 112). The subjective sensation that the world is turning around suggests **vertigo**, which can be due to vestibular abnormalities (e.g. labyrinthitis).

Intermittent claudication

A history of claudication (pain in the calves when walking a predictable distance) suggests peripheral vascular disease causing an inadequate arterial blood supply to the affected muscles.

Fatigue

Fatigue is a common symptom of cardiac failure but there are many other causes of this symptom, including depression and hypothyroidism.

Risk factors for cardiac disease

1. *Ischaemic heart disease.* The most important risk factors for ischaemic heart disease are:
   (a) previous episodes of ischaemic heart disease
   (b) hypertension
   (c) hyperlipidaemia
   (d) smoking
   (e) a family history of coronary artery disease (first-degree relatives—siblings or parents—affected before the age of 60)
   (f) diabetes mellitus
   (g) obesity
   (h) male sex and old age
   (i) erectile dysfunction and peripheral vascular disease.
   A raised homocysteine level may be an important factor in patients with premature coronary artery disease.
2. *Valvular heart disease.* A history of rheumatic fever places patients at risk for rheumatic valvular heart disease (usually aortic and mitral stenosis or regurgitation). Valvular and cardiac abnormalities are a feature of certain inherited conditions. Marfan's syndrome can be a cause of valve disease (e.g. aortic regurgitation, mitral valve prolapse) and aortic disease (e.g. aortic dissection). Down syndrome is a cause of atrial septal defects (a hole in the atrium) and mitral and tricuspid valve abnormalities.
3. A family history of *cardiac muscle abnormalities.* Some forms of dilated cardiomyopathy, a cause of heart failure (p. 49), and cases of hypertrophic cardiomyopathy (see Table 4.5) are inherited conditions. The disease severity may differ in different families.
4. *Sudden death and cardiac arrhythmias.* Inherited abnormalities of cardiac ion transport are associated with an increased risk of sudden death, such as the long QT interval syndrome and the Brugada syndrome (right bundle branch block pattern with septal ST elevation on the electrocardiogram).

Treatment history

Always ask about current and past drug treatment, the cardiac surgical history and any history of coronary artery angioplasty or balloon valvotomy.

Social history

Social history is relevant for patients with a chronic illness and must be recorded. The availability of family and financial support is important for any patient with a serious illness and may affect issues such as how soon the patient can go home. Many cardiac conditions affect a patient's ability to work. Heavy physical work may not be possible following an infarct or valve surgery. Certain specific occupations (e.g. commercial flying or vehicle driving) are precluded in patients with certain heart diseases if there is an increased risk of syncope or sudden death.

Examination anatomy

The mechanical function of the heart results in movement that is often palpable (see Fig 4.11 on p. 54) and sometimes visible on the part of the chest that lies in front of it—the praecordium. The passage of blood through the heart and its valves (see Figs 4.1 and 4.2) and on into the great vessels of the body produces many interesting sounds and causes pulsation in arteries and movement in veins in remote parts of the body. Signs of cardiac disease may be found by examining the praecordium and the many accessible arteries and veins of the body (see Fig 4.3).

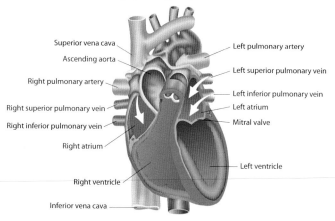

Superior vena cava
Ascending aorta
Right pulmonary artery
Right superior pulmonary vein
Right inferior pulmonary vein
Right atrium
Right ventricle
Inferior vena cava

Left pulmonary artery
Left superior pulmonary vein
Left inferior pulmonary vein
Left atrium
Mitral valve
Left ventricle

(a) Early diastole—ventricles begin to relax

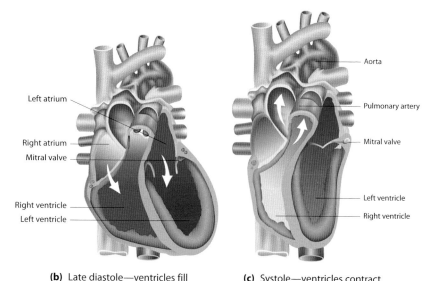

Left atrium
Right atrium
Mitral valve
Right ventricle
Left ventricle

(b) Late diastole—ventricles fill

Aorta
Pulmonary artery
Mitral valve
Left ventricle
Right ventricle

(c) Systole—ventricles contract

Figure 4.1 The cardiac cycle

(a)   **(b)**

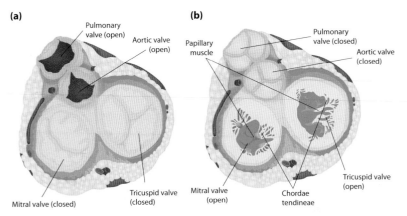

Figure 4.2 The cardiac valves in **(a)** systole and **(b)** diastole

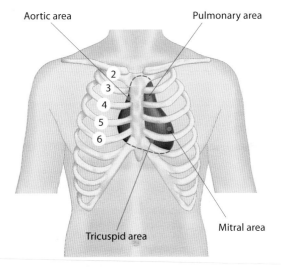

Figure 4.3 Surface anatomy of the heart

Examining the heart

Examination of the cardiovascular system usually begins with the peripheral signs of heart and vascular disease (namely, the radial pulse, blood pressure, and jugular venous pressure or JVP). These are described later in the chapter.

It is important to begin with the patient lying in bed with enough pillows to support him or her at 45° (see Fig 4.4). In this position the chest is easily accessible and this is the usual position in which the JVP is assessed (p. 58).

The praecordium should be examined anteriorly by inspection, palpation and auscultation.

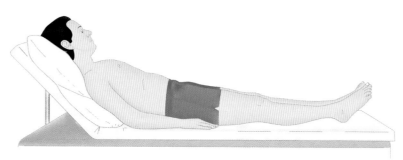

Figure 4.4 Position the patient at a 45° angle

Inspection

You will be looking (1) at the chest wall for scars and lumps and (2) for the apex beat (visible contraction of the left ventricle during systole).

Inspect first for **scars**. Previous cardiac operations will have left scars on the chest wall. Coronary artery and valve surgery are usually performed through a median sternotomy incision and a scar will be visible extending from just below the suprasternal notch to the xiphisternum.

Another surgical 'abnormality' is a **pacemaker box**. This box is usually placed under the right or left pectoral muscle, is easily palpable and obviously metallic.

The **apex beat** (see Fig 4.5) may be visible as a flickering movement of a small area (about 2 cm) of the skin of the chest wall between two ribs. It is caused by the twisting or wringing movement that occurs with ventricular systole (contraction). Its normal position is in the fifth left intercostal space 1 cm medial to the mid-clavicular line (see Fig 4.5).

Palpation

You will be trying to feel for:
1. the apex beat
2. thrills (palpable murmurs)
3. other impulses.

Count down the number of interspaces to where the apex beat is palpable (see Fig 4.5). The first palpable rib interspace is the second. The position of the apex beat is defined as the most lateral and inferior point at which the palpating fingers are raised with each systole. An apex beat displaced laterally or inferiorly, or both, usually indicates enlargement of the heart, but may occasionally be due to chest wall deformity, or pleural or pulmonary disease.

The normal apex beat gently lifts the palpating fingers. Try to decide whether the apex beat is normal or abnormal.
1. The **dyskinetic** apex beat feels uncoordinated and large. It is usually due to left ventricular dysfunction (e.g. previous anterior myocardial infarction or dilated cardiomyopathy).
2. The **volume-loaded** (hyperkinetic or diastolic overloaded) apex beat is a coordinated impulse felt over a larger area than normal in the

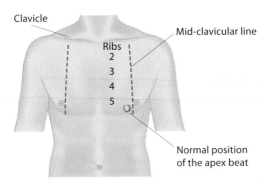

Figure 4.5 Finding the apex beat

praecordium and is usually the result of left ventricular dilatation (e.g. due to aortic regurgitation).

3. The **pressure-loaded** (hyperdynamic or systolic overloaded) apex beat is a forceful and sustained impulse. This occurs with aortic stenosis or hypertension.

In about 50% of people the apex beat is not palpable. This is most often due to a thick chest wall, emphysema, pericardial effusion, shock (or death) and very rarely to dextrocardia (where there is inversion of the heart and great vessels). The apex beat will be palpable to the right of the sternum in many cases of dextrocardia.

Turbulent blood flow, which is what causes cardiac murmurs on auscultation, may sometimes be palpable. These palpable murmurs are called **thrills**. The praecordium should be systematically palpated for thrills with the flat of the hand (palm side), first over the apex and left sternal edge, and then over the base of the heart (this is the upper part of the chest and includes the aortic and pulmonary areas; see Fig 4.6).

Apical thrills can be more easily felt with the patient rolled over to the left side (the left lateral position), because this brings the apex closer to the chest wall. Thrills may also be palpable over the **base of the heart**. These may be at a maximum over the pulmonary or aortic areas, depending on the underlying cause, and are best felt with the patient sitting up, leaning forward and in full expiration. In this position the base of the heart is moved closer to the chest wall. A thrill that coincides in time with the apex beat is called a **systolic thrill**, while one that does not coincide with the apex beat is called a **diastolic thrill**.

The presence of a thrill usually means there is a significant abnormality of the heart and that the associated murmur is not an **innocent** (normal variation) murmur.

Feel also for a **parasternal impulse**. The heel of the hand rests just to the left of the sternum with the fingers lifted slightly off the chest. In cases of right ventricular enlargement or severe left atrial enlargement, where the right ventricle is pushed anteriorly, the heel of the hand is lifted off the chest wall with each systole.

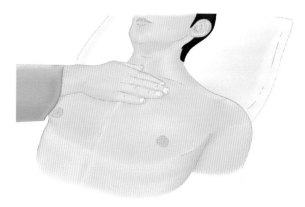

Figure 4.6 Palpating the base of the heart for palpable murmurs (thrills)

Palpation with the fingers over the pulmonary area (second left intercostal space) may reveal the *palpable tap of pulmonary valve closure (P2)* in cases of pulmonary hypertension.

Auscultation

You will be listening in each area of the heart for:

1. heart sounds (first and second)
2. extra heart sounds (third and fourth)
3. additional sounds (e.g. snaps, clicks or prosthetic heart sounds)
4. murmurs (which you will need to time, determine the area of greatest intensity, assess loudness and pitch, and, if indicated, perform dynamic manoeuvres)
5. rubs.

Auscultation of the heart traditionally begins in the **mitral area** (see Fig 4.7) with the **bell** of the stethoscope. The bell applied lightly to the chest wall better amplifies low-pitched sounds, such as the murmur of mitral stenosis (see Fig 4.8). Next listen in the mitral area with the **diaphragm** of the stethoscope, which best reproduces higher-pitched sounds, such as the systolic murmur of mitral regurgitation. Some newer stethoscopes reproduce the effect of the bell when the auscultator presses the diaphragm lightly on the chest and of the diaphragm when it is applied more firmly. This is convenient but deprives the clinician of a rotating stethoscope head to manipulate at times of worry. Now place the stethoscope in the tricuspid area (fifth left intercostal space) and listen with the diaphragm. Next inch up the left sternal edge to the pulmonary (second left intercostal space) and aortic (second right intercostal space) areas, again listening carefully in each position with the diaphragm.

Auscultation of the normal heart reveals two sounds called, not surprisingly, the first and second heart sounds. The **first heart sound (S1)** has two components: mitral valve closure and tricuspid valve closure. Mitral valve closure occurs slightly before that of the tricuspid valve, but usually

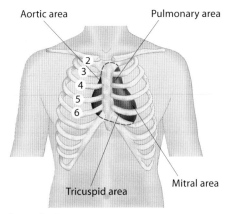

Figure 4.7 Areas of auscultation

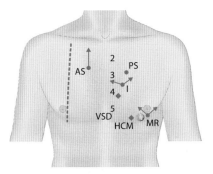

(a) Systolic murmurs

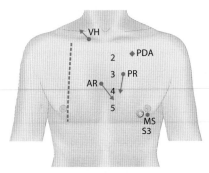

(b) Diastolic and continuous murmurs, and diastolic sounds

AS = aortic stenosis	**PR** = pulmonary regurgitation
PS = pulmonary stenosis	**AR** = aortic regurgitation
MR = mitral regurgitation	**MS** = mitral stenosis
VSD = ventricular septal defect	**S3** = third heart sound
HCM = hypertrophic cardiomyopathy	**VH** = venous hum
PDA = patent ductus arteriosus	**I** = innocent

Figure 4.8 Radiation and sites of maximum intensity of heart sounds and murmurs

only one sound is audible. The first heart sound indicates the beginning of ventricular contraction (systole); ventricular relaxation is called diastole.

The **second heart sound (S2)** at the apex is generally softer, shorter and higher pitched than the first (see Fig 4.9). It marks the end of systole and is made up of sounds from aortic and pulmonary valve closures. In normal cases, because of lower pressure in the pulmonary circulation compared with the aorta, closure of the pulmonary valve is later than that of the aortic valve. These components are usually sufficiently separated in time so that **splitting** of the second heart sound is audible and is best appreciated in the pulmonary area and along the left sternal edge. Pulmonary valve closure is further delayed with inspiration because of increased venous return to the right ventricle, and thus splitting of the second heart sound is **wider on inspiration**. The second heart sound marks the beginning of diastole, which is usually longer than systole.

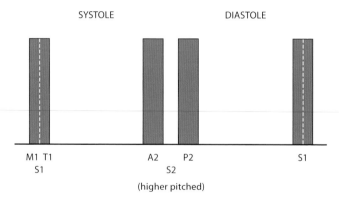

SYSTOLE   DIASTOLE

M1 T1   A2   P2   S1
S1   S2
(higher pitched)

S1 = first heart sound; S2 = second heart sound;
M1 = mitral component of S1; T1 = tricuspid component of S1;
A2 = aortic component of S2; P2 = pulmonary component of S2.

Figure 4.9 Normal heart sounds

It can be difficult to decide which heart sound is which. Palpation of the carotid pulsation in the neck will indicate the timing of systole and enable the heart sounds to be more easily distinguished.

Abnormalities of the heart sounds

Alterations in intensity

The first heart sound is **loud** when the mitral or tricuspid valve cups remain widely open at the end of diastole and shut forcefully with the onset of ventricular systole (see Fig 4.10). This occurs in mitral stenosis where the valve orifice has become narrowed, usually as a result of scarring of the leaflets from rheumatic fever. A **soft** first heart sound can be due to failure of the leaflets to coapt normally (as in mitral regurgitation where blood leaks back from the left ventricle into the left atrium during systole—this used to be called mitral incompetence or insufficiency).

The second heart sound may have a **loud aortic component (A2)** in patients with systemic hypertension. The **pulmonary component of the second heart sound (P2)** is loud in pulmonary hypertension, where the valve closure is forceful because of the high pulmonary pressure. A **soft A2** will be found when the aortic valve is calcified and leaflet movement is reduced, and in aortic regurgitation when the leaflets cannot coapt.

Splitting
Splitting of the first heart sound (see Fig 4.10) is usually not detectable clinically; however, when it occurs it is most often due to complete right bundle branch block (a cardiac conduction abnormality).

Increased normal splitting (wider on inspiration) of the second heart sound occurs when there is any delay in right ventricular emptying, as in right bundle branch block (delayed right ventricular depolarisation) or pulmonary stenosis (delayed right ventricular ejection).

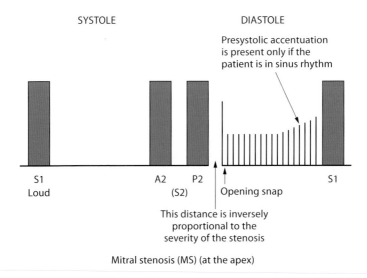

Mitral stenosis (MS) (at the apex)

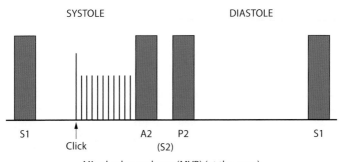

Mitral valve prolapse (MVP) (at the apex)

Figure 4.10 Heart sounds, clicks, snaps and splitting   *continued*

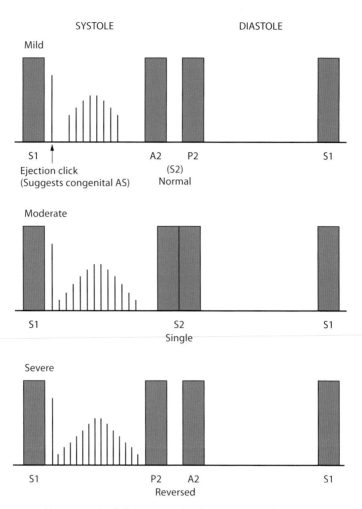

Figure 4.10 Heart sounds, clicks, snaps and splitting *continued*

In the case of **fixed splitting**, the normal respiratory variation is absent and splitting tends to be wide. This is caused by an atrial septal defect where equalisation of volume loads between the two atria occurs through the defect.

Extra heart sounds

The **third heart sound (S3)** is a low-pitched, mid-diastolic sound that is best appreciated by listening for the characteristic triple cadence of the cardiac rhythm. It has been likened (not unreasonably) to the sound of a galloping horse and is often called a gallop rhythm. It can be physiological in pregnancy. Otherwise, it is an important sign of left ventricular failure (see box below) but may also occur in aortic regurgitation or mitral regurgitation.

Signs of cardiac failure (in approximate order of helpfulness)

Right heart
Right ventricular third heart sound
Elevated jugular venous pressure
Signs of tricuspid regurgitation—large v waves, pulsatile liver
Peripheral oedema
Ascites

Left heart
Third heart sound
Displaced and dyskinetic apex beat
Bilateral basal inspiratory crackles (medium or coarse)
Dyspnoea and especially orthopnoea (a symptom and a sign)
Pleural effusion (left or bilateral)

The **fourth heart sound (S4)** is a late diastolic sound that is slightly more high-pitched than the S3. Again, this is responsible for the impression of a triple (gallop) rhythm. It is never physiological and is most often due to systemic hypertension (p. 29). It cannot be present if the patient has atrial fibrillation (p. 53).

Additional sounds
An **opening snap** is a high-pitched sound that occurs in mitral stenosis at a variable distance after S2 (see Fig 4.10). It is due to the sudden opening of the mitral valve and is followed by the diastolic murmur of mitral stenosis. It is best heard at the lower left sternal edge with the diaphragm of the stethoscope. Use of the term *opening snap* implies the diagnosis of mitral stenosis (or the very uncommon tricuspid stenosis).

A **systolic ejection click** is an early systolic, high-pitched sound heard over the aortic or pulmonary area, which may occur in cases of congenital aortic or pulmonary stenosis where the valve remains mobile; it is followed by the systolic ejection murmur of aortic or pulmonary stenosis.

A **non-ejection systolic click** is a high-pitched sound heard during systole and is best appreciated at the mitral area. It is a common finding. It may be followed by a systolic murmur. The click may be due to prolapse of one or both redundant mitral valve leaflets during systole.

Mechanical prosthetic heart valves produce characteristic crisp metallic sounds.

Murmurs of the heart
The correct diagnosis of a murmur depends on the synthesis of findings made at the praecordium (apex beat, thrills etc), the noise itself and peripheral signs.

Timing
See Table 4.3. **Systolic murmurs** (which occur during ventricular systole) may be pansystolic, ejection (mid-) systolic or late systolic.

The **pansystolic murmur** extends throughout systole, beginning with the first heart sound, then going right up to the second heart sound. Causes of

Table 4.3 Cardiac murmurs

Timing	Lesion	Maximum intensity
Pansystolic	Mitral regurgitation	Apex
	Tricuspid regurgitation	Lower left sternal edge
	Ventricular septal defect	Lower left sternal edge
Mid-systolic	Aortic stenosis	Base (aortic area)
	Pulmonary stenosis	Base (pulmonary area)
	Hypertrophic cardiomyopathy	Lower left sternal edge
	Pulmonary flow murmur of an atrial septal defect	Pulmonary area
Late systolic	Mitral valve prolapse	Apex
	Papillary muscle dysfunction (due usually to ischaemia or hypertrophic cardiomyopathy)	Apex
Early diastolic	Aortic regurgitation	Lower left sternal edge
	Pulmonary regurgitation	Left sternal edge
Mid-diastolic	Mitral stenosis	Apex
	Tricuspid stenosis	Right lower sternal edge
Presystolic	Mitral stenosis	Apex
	Tricuspid stenosis	Right lower sternal edge
	Atrial myxoma	Apex
Continuous	Patent ductus arteriosus	Below left clavicle
	Arteriovenous fistula (coronary artery, pulmonary, systemic)	Left sternal edge
	Aorto-pulmonary connection	Left sternal edge
	Venous hum (abolished by ipsilateral internal jugular vein compression)	Supraclavicular fossa
	Rupture of sinus of Valsalva into right ventricle or atrium	Left sternal edge

Note: The combined murmurs of aortic stenosis and aortic regurgitation, or mitral stenosis and mitral regurgitation, may sound as if they fill the entire cardiac cycle but are not continuous murmurs by definition.

pansystolic murmurs include some types of mitral regurgitation, tricuspid regurgitation and ventricular septal defect.

An **ejection (mid-) systolic** murmur does not begin right at the first heart sound; its intensity is greatest in mid-systole or later and wanes again late in systole. This is described as a crescendo–decrescendo murmur. These murmurs are usually caused by turbulent flow through the aortic or pulmonary valve orifices, or by greatly increased flow through a normal-sized orifice or outflow tract.

If a murmur is **late systolic**, a gap can be distinguished between the first heart sound and the murmur which then continues right up to the second heart sound. This is typical of mitral valve prolapse or papillary muscle dysfunction where mitral regurgitation begins in mid-systole.

Diastolic murmurs occur during ventricular diastole. **Early diastolic murmurs** begin immediately with the second heart sound and have a decrescendo quality (i.e. they are loudest at the beginning and extend for a variable distance into diastole). Early diastolic murmurs are typically high-pitched and are due to regurgitation through a leaking aortic or (less commonly) pulmonary valve.

Mid-diastolic murmurs begin later in diastole and may be short or extend right up to the first heart sound. They have a much lower pitched quality than early diastolic murmurs. They are due to impaired flow during ventricular filling and can be caused by mitral stenosis where the valve is narrowed.

Presystolic murmurs may be heard when atrial systole increases blood flow across the valve just before the first heart sound. They are an extension of the mid-diastolic murmurs of mitral stenosis and tricuspid stenosis, and are absent in patients who are in atrial fibrillation (because atrial systole is lost).

Continuous murmurs extend throughout systole and diastole. They are produced when a communication exists between two parts of the circulation with a permanent pressure gradient so that blood flow occurs continuously (e.g. patent (persistent) ductus arteriosus). They should be distinguished from combined systolic and diastolic murmurs (due, for example, to aortic stenosis and aortic regurgitation).

A **pericardial friction rub** is a superficial scratching sound; there may be up to three distinct components occurring at any time during the cardiac cycle. They are not confined to systole or diastole. A rub is caused by movement of inflamed pericardial surfaces. The sound can vary with respiration and posture; it is often louder when the patient is sitting up and breathing out. It tends to come and go. Its presence cannot exclude a significant pericardial fluid collection, since the pericardial surfaces may still be opposed at points of reflection and where the fluid is loculated.

Area of greatest intensity (Fig 4.8)
Unfortunately the place on the praecordium where a murmur is loudest is not a very reliable guide to its origin. For example, the murmur of mitral regurgitation, although clearly audible at the apex, may be heard widely over the praecordium and even right up into the aortic area or over the back. Conduction of an ejection systolic murmur up into the carotid arteries,

however, suggests that this arises from the aortic valve. The murmur of a ventricular septal defect is loudest in the right parasternal area and is not well heard at the base of the heart or at the apex. This helps distinguish it from the murmurs of aortic stenosis and mitral regurgitation, respectively.

Loudness and pitch

The loudness of the murmur may not be helpful in deciding the severity of the valve lesion. Harshness is perhaps a better guide. Changes in the loudness, however, are very important. Murmurs are usually graded according to loudness. Cardiologists most often use a classification with six grades:

- **grade 1/6:** very soft and audible only in ideal listening conditions
- **grade 2/6:** soft, but can be detected almost immediately by an experienced auscultator
- **grade 3/6:** moderate; there is no thrill
- **grade 4/6:** loud; thrill just palpable
- **grade 5/6:** very loud; thrill easily palpable
- **grade 6/6:** very, very loud (and very rare); can be heard even without placing the stethoscope on the chest.

Dynamic manoeuvres

1. *Respiration.* Listen to the murmur as the patient breathes deeply in and out. Murmurs that arise on the right side of the heart tend to be louder during inspiration because this increases venous return and therefore blood flow to the right side of the heart.
2. *Valsalva manoeuvre.* This is a forceful expiration against a closed glottis. The manoeuvre provokes a complicated series of haemodynamic responses in four phases:
   - In phase 1 there is a transient increase in blood pressure caused by straining and the rise in intrathoracic pressure.
   - In phase 2 systolic blood pressure and pulse pressure decrease and there is an increase in the heart rate. This is due to a reduction in venous return to the heart and a fall in stroke volume.
   - In phase 3 there is the initial release of straining, which causes a brief further fall in blood pressure due to the fall in intrathoracic pressure.
   - In phase 4 there is an overshoot of blood pressure associated with bradycardia.

   Ask the patient to breathe in, hold his or her nose with the fingers, close the mouth, breathe out hard and completely so as to pop the eardrums, and hold this for as long as possible. Listen over the left sternal edge during this manoeuvre for changes in the systolic murmur of hypertrophic cardiomyopathy, and over the apex for changes when mitral valve prolapse is suspected. The reduction in left ventricular volume that occurs before the breath is released causes the murmur of hypertrophic cardiomyopathy to become louder and the murmur and click of mitral valve prolapse to occur earlier. All other murmurs become softer as stroke volume is reduced.

3. *Exercise.* If mitral stenosis is suspected but the diastolic murmur is difficult to hear, it is helpful to exercise the patient by getting him or her to sit up and down a number of times. Get the patient then to lie quickly on the left side and listen at the apex with the bell.

The peripheral signs of heart disease

General appearance

Note the patient's *general state of health.* Look to see whether the patient has *rapid and laboured respiration,* suggesting dyspnoea, which is both a symptom and a sign. Dyspnoea may be present as the patient undresses or even at rest. Look for *cachexia*—that is, severe loss of weight and muscle wasting. This is commonly caused by malignant disease, but severe cardiac failure may also produce this appearance (cardiac cachexia).

The hands

Pick up the right hand, then the left. Look for **peripheral cyanosis**, which is blue discolouration of the fingers, toes and other peripheral parts of the body. Look at the nails from the side for **clubbing** (see Fig 3.3). This is an increase in the soft tissue of the distal part of the fingers or toes, and occurs in cyanotic congenital heart disease (see Table 3.2).

Also look for **splinter haemorrhages** in the nail beds. These are linear haemorrhages lying parallel to the long axis of the nail (see Fig 3.3). They are most often due to trauma, particularly in manual workers. However, an important cause is infective endocarditis, which is a bacterial (or less commonly a fungal) infection of the heart valves or part of the endocardium.

Tendon xanthomata are yellow or orange deposits of lipid in the tendons, including those of the hand and arm. They occur in hyperlipidaemia.

The arterial pulse

The following observations should be made at the radial pulse (see Fig 4.11):
1. rate of pulse
2. rhythm
3. presence or absence of delay of the femoral pulse compared with the radial pulse (radiofemoral delay; see Fig 4.12). See Table 4.4.

Rate of pulse

The pulse rate can be counted over 30 seconds and multiplied by two. The normal resting heart rate in adults is between 60 and 100 beats per minute. Bradycardia is defined as a heart rate less than 60 beats per minute. Tachycardia is defined as a heart rate over 100 beats per minute.

Rhythm

The rhythm of the pulse can be regular or **irregular**. An irregular rhythm can be completely *irregular with no pattern*; this is usually due to atrial fibrillation, which occurs when coordinated contraction of the atria is lost and the ventricles beat irregularly and usually fast. The pulse rate is then usually rapid (greater than 120 beats per minute) unless the patient is being treated with drugs to slow it down. An irregularly irregular pulse can occasionally be caused by frequent, irregularly occurring supraventricular or ventricular ectopic beats (extra-systoles). An irregular rhythm can also be *regularly irregular*. For example, in sinus arrhythmia the pulse rate increases with each inspiration and decreases with each expiration. This is normal.

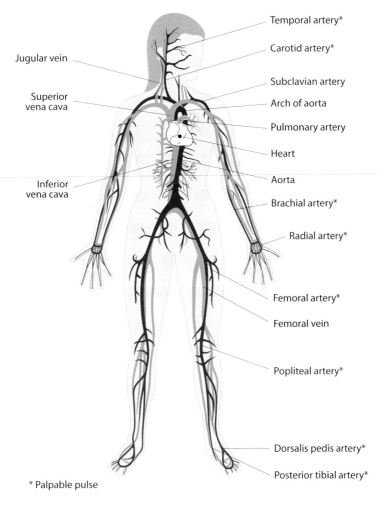

Temporal artery*
Carotid artery*
Jugular vein
Subclavian artery
Superior vena cava
Arch of aorta
Pulmonary artery
Heart
Inferior vena cava
Aorta
Brachial artery*
Radial artery*
Femoral artery*
Femoral vein
Popliteal artery*
Dorsalis pedis artery*
Posterior tibial artery*

* Palpable pulse

Figure 4.11 The palpable arteries (pulses)

Table 4.4 The character of the arterial pulse

Type of pulse	Cause(s)
Anacrotic Small volume, slow uptake, notched wave on upstroke	Aortic stenosis
Plateau Slow upstroke	Aortic stenosis
Bisferiens Anacrotic and collapsing	Aortic stenosis and regurgitation
Collapsing	Aortic regurgitation Hyperdynamic circulation Patent ductus arteriosus Peripheral arteriovenous fistula Arteriosclerotic aorta (elderly patients in particular)
Small volume	Aortic stenosis Pericardial effusion
Pulsus paradoxus	Tamponade or severe asthma

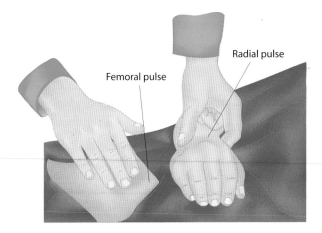

Figure 4.12 Feeling for radiofemoral delay

Character and volume

The character and volume of the pulse are better assessed from palpation of the brachial or carotid arteries. However, the collapsing (bounding) pulse of aortic regurgitation may be readily apparent at the wrist.

The blood pressure

The systolic blood pressure (see p. 27) is the peak pressure that occurs in the artery following ventricular systole, and the diastolic blood pressure is the level to which the arterial blood pressure falls during ventricular diastole.

High blood pressure

The risk of adverse outcome increases as the blood pressure rises above normal. **Malignant hypertension** is marked hypertension (usually the diastolic is >120 mmHg) with changes on fundoscopy (haemorrhages, exudates and papilloedema; p. 148).

Postural blood pressure

The blood pressure should routinely be taken with the patient lying and standing (or sitting). A fall in blood pressure of more than 15 mmHg in systolic blood pressure or 10 mmHg in diastolic blood pressure on standing is abnormal and is called *postural hypotension*. It may not be associated with symptoms.

Changes with respiration: pulsus paradoxus

A **fall in systolic blood** pressure of up to 10 mmHg occurs normally during inspiration. Exaggeration of this response—a fall of more than 10 mmHg—is an important sign of pericardial tamponade (rapid accumulation of fluid in the pericardial space) or severe asthma. It is detected by lowering the cuff pressure slowly (p. 29).

The face

Xanthelasma are intracutaneous yellow cholesterol deposits around the eyes and are relatively common. These may be a normal variant or may indicate hyperlipidaemia.

In the mouth, use a torch to see whether there is a **high arched palate**. This occurs in *Marfan's syndrome*, a condition that is associated with congenital heart disease, including aortic regurgitation secondary to aortic dilatation, and also with mitral regurgitation due to mitral valve prolapse. Look for **diseased teeth** as they can be a source of organisms responsible for infective endocarditis. Look at the tongue and lips for **central cyanosis**, which refers to a blue discolouration from an abnormal amount of deoxygenated haemoglobin in parts of the body with a good circulation.

The neck

Useful information about cardiac function is available in most patients' necks. Arterial (carotid) and venous (jugular) pulsations should be examined.

1. *Carotid arteries.* The carotid pulse can be felt medial to the sternomastoid muscle by applying slight posterior and medial pressure with the middle and forefingers (see Fig 4.13). Evaluation of the amplitude, shape and volume of the pulse is used to help in the diagnosis of various underlying cardiac diseases and in assessing their severity. Important carotid pulse abnormalities are described in Table 4.4.

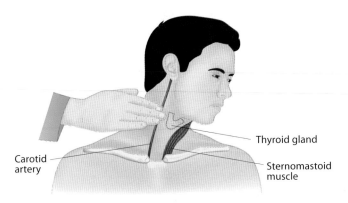

Thyroid gland

Carotid
artery

Sternomastoid
muscle

Figure 4.13 Feeling the carotid pulse

2. *Jugular venous pressure (JVP).* The internal jugular vein runs a direct course to the right atrium (see Fig 4.14). By convention, the *sternal angle* is taken as the zero point, and the maximum height of pulsations in the internal jugular vein, which are visible above the sternal angle when the patient is at 45°, can be measured in centimetres.

The jugular venous pulsation can be distinguished from the arterial pulse because it: (1) is visible but not palpable; (2) has a complex wave form, usually seen to flicker twice with each cardiac cycle (if the patient is in sinus rhythm); (3) moves on respiration—normally the JVP decreases on inspiration; and (4) is at first obliterated and then filled from above when light pressure is applied at the base of the neck.

The JVP must be assessed for **height** and **character**. When the JVP is more than 3 cm above the zero point, the right heart filling pressure is raised. This is a sign of right ventricular failure or volume overload.

There are two positive waves in the normal JVP. The first wave is called the **a wave** and coincides with right atrial systole. It is due to atrial contraction. The a wave also coincides with the first heart sound and precedes the carotid pulsation. The second impulse is called the **v wave** and is due to atrial filling in the period when the tricuspid valve remains closed during ventricular systole (see Fig 4.14).

Any condition in which right ventricular filling is limited (e.g. constrictive pericarditis, cardiac tamponade or right ventricular infarction) can cause elevation of the venous pressure, which is more marked on inspiration when venous return to the heart increases. This *rise in the JVP on inspiration,* called **Kussmaul's sign,** is the opposite of what normally happens. The sign is best elicited with the patient sitting up at 90° and breathing quietly through the mouth.

Cannon a waves occur when the right atrium contracts against the closed tricuspid valve. This is usually due to cardiac electrical abnormalities that have resulted in dissociation of atrial and ventricular contraction (e.g. complete heart block). **Large v waves** occur in tricuspid regurgitation.

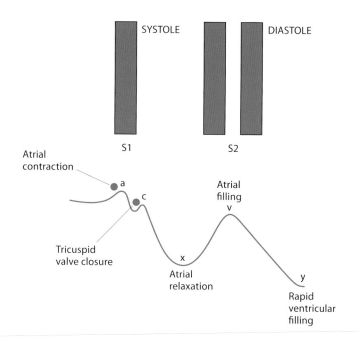

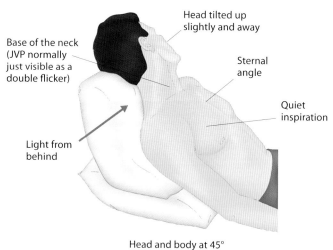

Figure 4.14 The jugular venous pressure

The **abdominojugular reflux test** can be performed as a test of right ventricular failure if the JVP is not raised. Apply steady pressure over the right upper or middle abdomen for 10 seconds. There may be a brief rise in the JVP to over 4 cm. If this is sustained for the duration of the compression, the test is positive. This is a good sign of ventricular failure.

The back

Percussion and auscultation of the lung bases (Ch 5) are also part of the cardiovascular examination. Signs of cardiac failure may be detected in the lungs; in particular, late or pan-inspiratory crackles or a pleural effusion (usually left-sided) may be present. Remember that basal crackles are common and not always due to cardiac failure. While the patient is sitting up, feel for *pitting oedema of the sacrum* (see below), which occurs in severe right heart failure, especially in patients who have been in bed.

The abdomen

Lay the patient down flat (on one pillow) and examine the abdomen (Ch 6). The liver may become enlarged and tender due to hepatic venous congestion in patients with right ventricular failure. In severe cases this may be accompanied by ascites (peritoneal fluid).

The lower limbs

Examine both femoral arteries (found by feeling in the inguinal crease midway between the anterior superior iliac spine and the pubic tubercle) (p. 60), and then all the arteries of the legs (see Fig 4.15): the popliteal (behind the knee), posterior tibial (under the medial malleolus) and dorsalis pedis (on the forefoot) on both sides.

Palpate the distal shaft of the tibia for oedema by compressing the area gently for at least 15 seconds with the thumb. If **pitting oedema** is present, a little pit will appear in the shape of your thumb and refill only gradually.

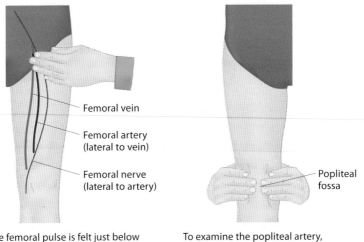

Femoral vein

Femoral artery
(lateral to vein)

Femoral nerve
(lateral to artery)

Popliteal
fossa

The femoral pulse is felt just below the inguinal ligament midway between the anterior superior iliac crest and the symphysis pubis

To examine the popliteal artery, the leg is flexed to relax the hamstrings, and firm compression is applied against the lower end of the tibia

(a) Left leg anterior

(b) Left leg posterior

Figure 4.15 Sites of the peripheral pulses

continued

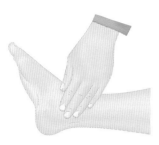
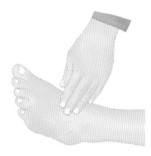

The posterior tibial artery is felt just behind the tip of the medial malleolus

The dorsalis pedis is felt at the proximal end of the first intermetatarsal space

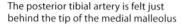

Figure 4.15 Sites of the peripheral pulses *continued*

Leg ulcers (which are typically on the medial side of the lower third of the leg above the medial malleolus when due to venous disease) and **varicose veins** should be noted. If varicose veins are present, the site of **venous valvular incompetence** should be determined. Examine for long saphenous incompetence as follows:

1. *Cough impulse test.* After standing the patient up, palpate just below the fossa ovalis (where the vein passes to join the femoral vein), which is 4 cm below and 4 cm lateral to the pubic tubercle (a prominent, forward-projecting, round nodule of bone on the upper medial portion of the pubis). Ask the patient to cough. Feel for an impulse (thrill). Look also for a **saphena varix** (dilatation of the vein that produces a swelling in the fossa ovalis, which, unlike a femoral hernia, disappears when the patient lies down).
2. *Trendelenburg test.* After lying the patient down, elevate the patient's leg to empty the veins. Then compress the upper end of the vein in the groin with your hand and stand the patient up; normally, if little or no filling occurs until the groin pressure is released, sapheno-femoral valve incompetence is present and the test is positive. If filling occurs before the pressure is released, incompetent veins are in the thigh or calf.

Deep venous thrombosis

The presence of calf pain at rest should suggest the possibility of deep venous thrombosis. Examine for swelling of the affected calf and dilated superficial veins. Tenderness and warmth may be present on palpation. These signs have, unfortunately, not been shown to be sensitive or specific for this condition.

The cardiovascular examination OSCE: hints panel

This OSCE is usually centred around the diagnosis of common cardiac murmurs, signs of heart failure or peripheral vascular disease. The examiner will usually direct you to a region to be examined.

Always introduce yourself to the patient first and ask permission to perform an examination. Try to synthesise the findings as you go along.

1   **This patient has been breathless on exertion and has a murmur. Please examine his praecordium.**
   (a) If necessary ask the patient to uncover his chest and stand back for a moment to look for breathlessness at rest, and cyanosis.
   (b) Look at the patient's chest for surgical scars or deformity. Look for the apex beat.
   (c) Feel for the apex beat, thrills and a parasternal impulse (p. 43).
   (d) Listen with the bell and then the diaphragm at the apex. Listen with the diaphragm at the left sternal edge and at the base of the heart.
   (e) Sit the patient up and listen at the left sternal edge and at the base with the patient in deep expiration.
   (f) Listen over the carotids.
   (g) If you are confident of the diagnosis, tell the examiner, e.g. 'There is evidence this patient has aortic stenosis of moderate severity'. Then describe the physical findings. If you are unsure, describe the abnormal findings before committing to any diagnosis.

2   **This woman has been breathless on exertion and wakes breathless at night. Please examine her.**
   (a) Ask the patient to undress if necessary but leave a towel or part of a gown across her breasts.
   (b) Stand back to look for obvious breathlessness due to cardiac failure.
   (c) Look at the jugular venous pressure.
   (d) Look at the praecordium for the apex beat, scars etc.
   (e) Make a careful attempt to find and assess the apex beat. Feel for thrills and a parasternal impulse.
   (f) Auscultate for murmurs and a gallop rhythm.
   (g) Examine the chest posteriorly and look for peripheral oedema.
   (h) Synthesise and present your findings.

3   **This man is a smoker and has pains in his calves when he walks. Please examine his legs.**
   (a) Ask the patient to uncover his legs to at least the mid thighs.
   (b) Stand back for a general inspection; note dyspnoea, cyanosis and nicotine staining of the fingers.
   (c) Look at the legs for missing toes. Note cyanosis, hair loss over the lower legs or feet, and skin and calf muscle atrophy.
   (d) Examine the peripheral pulses, starting with the feet and working back to the femorals if distal pulses are reduced or absent.
   (e) Look for the scars of previous peripheral bypass operations. These are usually seen extending longitudinally across the femoral artery.
   (f) Synthesise and present your findings.

4   **This man has swelling of his ankles. Please examine his legs.**
   (a) Ask the patient to uncover his legs, using a towel to cover his groin. Lay him flat if possible.
   (b) Stand back to look for peripheral oedema, and its extent, abdominal distension (ascites), dyspnoea and signs of chronic lung disease (p. 68).
   (c) Examine for pitting oedema and establish its upper level. Remember that it may involve the genitals and abdominal wall if severe.
   (d) Look for varicose veins.

(e) Examine the abdomen for ascites (p. 92), and feel the liver for enlargement and for signs of tricuspid regurgitation (liver pulsatile).
(f) Palpate for sacral oedema.
(g) Examine the heart and lungs.
(h) Synthesise and present your findings.

5 This man has developed central chest pain of sudden onset. Please examine him.

(a) Examine all relevant systems to narrow the differential diagnosis.
   (i) Examine the patient's pulses for arrhythmias.
   (ii) Take the patient's blood pressure.
   (iii) Look for signs of cardiac failure: JVP, oedema.
   (iv) Auscultate the heart for a gallop rhythm (heart failure) and a new murmur (e.g. papillary muscle rupture causing severe mitral regurgitation; signs of a ventricular septal defect post myocardial infarction).
   (v) Examine the chest wall for tenderness (costochondritis), and assess for any mediastinal shift (tension pneumothorax).
   (vi) Palpate the abdomen for tenderness (referred pain).
   (vii) Examine the back (referred pain).
(b) Synthesise and present your findings.

The cardiovascular system   hints for success

1 Ischaemic heart disease should be suspected from the history. When angina is stable, the pain or discomfort occurs with a predictable amount of exertion and is relieved by rest. A recent increase in the frequency or the occurrence of pain at rest suggests unstable angina.

2 Cardiac dyspnoea (i.e. breathlessness due to cardiac failure) is worse on exertion or when the patient lies flat (orthopnoea).

3 Ask about cardiac risk factors in any patient with suspected cardiac disease; for example, known high level of cholesterol and triglycerides, smoking, diabetes mellitus, family history of cardiac disease in first-degree relatives.

4 Pay particular attention when examining the cardiovascular system to the rate, rhythm and character of the pulse, the level of the blood pressure, elevation of the JVP, the position of the apex beat and the presence of the heart sounds, any extra sounds or murmurs.

5 The position and timing of cardiac murmurs give important clues about the underlying valve lesion.

6 The most useful cardiac signs of left ventricular failure are a third heart sound and a displaced and dyskinetic apex beat.

7 The diastolic murmur of aortic regurgitation is characteristic and has high diagnostic utility.

chapter 5

The chest

Chest: The trunk of the body, or cavity from the shoulders to the belly.

S Johnson, *A Dictionary of the English Language* (1755)

In this chapter, the symptoms and signs of lung disease are presented. The assessment begins with the history (concentrating in detail on the presenting symptoms). The chapter sets out the chest examination first, but the formal examination usually begins with an assessment of the peripheral signs of lung disease, as set out below.

The respiratory system assessment sequence

1 Presenting symptoms, e.g. dyspnoea, cough, wheeze, fever
2 Detailed questions about presenting symptoms (SOCRATES, p. 4)
3 Questions about previous lung problems and respiratory risk factors (e.g. smoking, occupation, pets)
4 Examination for peripheral signs of respiratory disease
5 Examination of the chest
6 Provisional and differential diagnosis

The respiratory history

Presenting symptoms (see Table 5.1)

Cough and sputum

Cough is a common presenting respiratory symptom. Ask about the duration, whether it is dry or productive (i.e. of sputum), whether it is associated with wheeze and whether the patient is taking any medications. Since the quality of the cough is important, ask the patient to describe the type of cough and to give a demonstration.

- A **cough of recent origin**, particularly if associated with fever and other symptoms of respiratory tract infection, may be due to acute bronchitis or pneumonia.
- A **chronic cough associated with wheezing** may be due to asthma; sometimes asthma can present with just cough alone.
- An **irritating chronic dry cough** can result from the reflux of acid into the oesophagus or the use of certain antihypertensive drugs (angiotensin-converting enzyme (ACE) inhibitors).

A change in the character of a chronic cough may indicate the development of a new and serious underlying problem (e.g. infection or lung cancer).

A large volume of **purulent** (yellow or green) **sputum** suggests the diagnosis of bronchiectasis or lobar pneumonia. **Foul-smelling, dark-coloured sputum** may indicate the presence of a lung abscess with anaerobic organisms. **Pink frothy secretions** from the trachea, which occur in pulmonary oedema, should not be confused with sputum. **Haemoptysis** (coughing up of blood) can be a sinister sign of lung disease and must always be investigated, because it may be due to carcinoma of the lung, pneumonia, tuberculosis, pulmonary infarction or bronchiectasis.

Table 5.1 The respiratory history: presenting symptoms
Major symptoms
Cough
Sputum
Haemoptysis
Dyspnoea (acute or chronic, progressive or paroxysmal)
Wheeze
Chest pain
Fever
Hoarseness

Dyspnoea

Careful questioning about the timing of onset, severity and pattern of dyspnoea is helpful in making the diagnosis. Dyspnoea that is *worse when the patient lies flat* or that *wakes the patient from sleep* is more likely to be due to cardiac failure than to a respiratory problem. *Exertional dyspnoea* associated with a sensation of chest tightness may be a presentation of angina. Patients with a history of smoking or occupational dust exposure often have a respiratory cause. The presence of fever or productive cough also points to a lung problem. In three cases out of four the cause of dyspnoea can be diagnosed from the history.

Dyspnoea can be graded from I to IV:
- class I—dyspnoea on heavy exertion
- class II—dyspnoea on moderate exertion
- class III—dyspnoea on minimal exertion
- class IV—dyspnoea at rest.

It may be more useful, however, to determine the amount of exertion that is actually needed to cause dyspnoea (i.e. the distance walked, or the number of steps climbed) or the patient's ability to perform daily tasks, such as dressing and washing.

Wheeze

A number of conditions can cause a continuous whistling noise during breathing (wheeze). These include *asthma, chronic obstructive pulmonary disease* (chronic obstructive airways disease) and *airway obstruction* by a foreign body or tumour.

Chest pain

Chest pain due to respiratory disease is characteristically *pleuritic* in nature (i.e. sharp and worse with deep inspiration and coughing).

Other presenting symptoms

Patients may occasionally present with episodes of **fever at night** (e.g. tuberculosis and pneumonia) or **hoarseness** (e.g. laryngitis, vocal cord tumour or recurrent laryngeal nerve palsy).

Patients with **obstructive sleep apnoea** (where airflow stops despite persistent respiratory efforts during sleep) typically present with daytime sleepiness (somnolence), chronic fatigue, morning headaches and personality disturbances. Very loud snoring may be reported by anyone within earshot.

Some patients respond to anxiety by increasing the rate and depth of their breathing. This is called **hyperventilation**. The resultant alkalosis may result in paraesthesia of the fingers and around the mouth, light-headedness, chest pain and a feeling of impending collapse. Anxiety (e.g. during a panic attack) can also make patients feel that they need to take deep breaths.

Past history

Always ask about any previous respiratory illness (including pneumonia, tuberculosis and exacerbations of chronic bronchitis) or abnormalities of the chest X-ray or computed tomography (CT) scan that have been previously reported to the patient.

Treatment

It is important to find out what drugs the patient is using, how often the drugs are taken and whether they are inhaled or swallowed. Almost every class of drug can produce lung toxicity. Examples include pulmonary embolism from use of the oral contraceptive pill, interstitial lung disease from cytotoxic agents, bronchospasm from beta-blockers or aspirin, and cough from ACE inhibitors.

Occupational history

Ask in some detail about possible exposure to *dusts* in mines and factories (e.g. asbestos, coal, silica, iron oxide, tin oxide, cotton, beryllium, titanium oxide, silver, nitrogen dioxide and anhydrides). Work or household exposure to *animals*, including birds, is also relevant (e.g. Q fever or psittacosis). Exposure to *mouldy hay*, humidifiers or air-conditioners may also result in lung disease (e.g. allergic alveolitis). Exposure to spray painting and wood dusts may provoke *occupational asthma*, which may typically resolve on weekends or on holidays.

Social history

A smoking history must be taken as a routine, because smoking is the major cause of chronic obstructive pulmonary disease and lung cancer. It is necessary to ask how many packets of cigarettes a day the patient has smoked and for how many years the patient has smoked. The number of packet years of smoking can be calculated from this information, but remember that cigarette packets often now contain more than the previous standard of 20 cigarettes.

Family history

A family history of asthma, cystic fibrosis or emphysema should be sought. Alpha$_1$-antitrypsin deficiency, for example, is an inherited disease associated with a family history of the development of emphysema in young middle-age.

Examination anatomy

The examination of the lungs makes more sense when the basic anatomy and function of the lungs and airways is kept in mind (see Figs 5.1 and 5.2). Always try to picture the structures that lie beneath the area of the chest being examined.

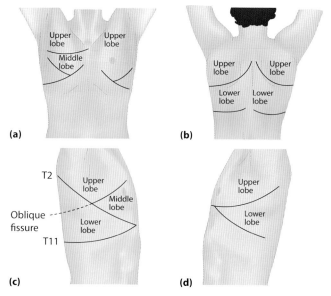

Figure 5.1 Lobes of the lung—surface markings
(a) Anterior **(b)** Posterior **(c)** Right lateral **(d)** Left lateral

5

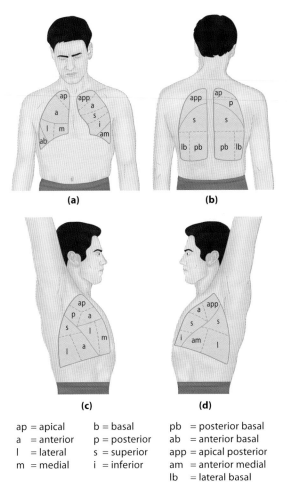

(a)   **(b)**

(c)   **(d)**

ap = apical   b = basal   pb = posterior basal
a = anterior   p = posterior   ab = anterior basal
l = lateral   s = superior   app = apical posterior
m = medial   i = inferior   am = anterior medial
                                  lb   = lateral basal

Figure 5.2 Surface markings of the segments of the lungs
(a) Anterior **(b)** Posterior **(c)** Right lateral **(d)** Left lateral

Examining the chest

Examination of the chest should include a search for signs of lung disease, chest wall abnormalities and examination of the female breasts (see Ch 10). The patient should be undressed to the waist and, if well enough, should sit over the edge of the bed.

General appearance

It is important to look for tachypnoea (a respiratory rate of more than 25 breaths per minute), use of the accessory muscles of respiration (sternomastoids, strap muscles and platysma, see Fig 5.3), cyanosis and a spontaneous cough.

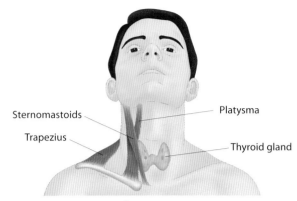

Figure 5.3 The accessory muscles of respiration

The chest

The chest should be examined anteriorly and posteriorly by **inspection**, **palpation**, **percussion** and **auscultation**. Compare the right and left sides during each part of the examination.

Inspection

The shape and symmetry of the chest

When the anteroposterior (AP) diameter is increased compared with the lateral diameter, the chest is described as **barrel-shaped** (see Fig 5.4(a)). An increase in the AP diameter indicates *hyperinflation*. **Kyphosis** refers to an exaggerated forward curvature of the spine, while **scoliosis** is lateral bowing (see Fig 5.4(b)). Severe thoracic kyphoscoliosis may reduce the lung capacity and increase the work of breathing. Other quite common varieties in chest shape include pectus excavatum and pectus carinatum (pigeon chest) (see Fig 5.4(c) and (d)).

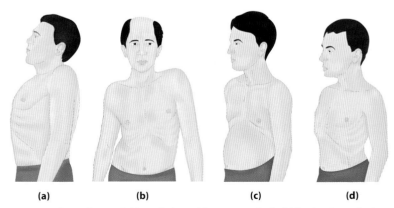

| (a) | (b) | (c) | (d) |

Figure 5.4 Chest shapes: **(a)** barrel-shaped (overexpanded); **(b)** kyphosis, scoliosis; **(c)** pectus excavatum and **(d)** pectus carinatum

Lesions of the chest wall

Look for **scars** from previous thoracic operations, or from chest drains inserted for a previous pneumothorax (often just below the clavicle) or pleural effusion (usually posterior and basal).

Radiotherapy for carcinoma of the lung or lymphoma may cause erythema and thickening of the skin over the irradiated area. There is a sharp demarcation between abnormal and normal skin.

Subcutaneous emphysema is a crackling sensation felt on palpating the skin of the chest or neck. It is caused by air tracking from the lungs and is usually due to a pneumothorax.

Prominent veins may be seen in patients with superior vena caval obstruction.

Movement of the chest wall

Look for **asymmetry** of chest wall movement anteriorly and posteriorly. Assessment of expansion of the **upper lobes** is best achieved by inspection from behind the patient, looking down at the clavicles during moderate respiration. The affected side will show delayed or decreased movement. For assessment of **lower lobe** expansion, the chest should be inspected posteriorly.

Reduced chest wall movement on one side may be due to localised pulmonary fibrosis, consolidation, collapse, pleural effusion or pneumothorax. *Bilateral reduction* of chest wall movement indicates a diffuse abnormality, such as chronic obstructive pulmonary disease or diffuse pulmonary fibrosis.

Palpation

Chest expansion

Place the hands firmly on the back of the chest wall with the fingers extending around the sides of the chest. The thumbs should almost meet in the middle line and should be lifted slightly off the chest so that they are free to move with respiration (see Fig 5.5). As the patient takes a big breath in, the thumbs should move apart symmetrically at least 5 cm. Reduced expansion on one side indicates a lesion of the lower lobe on that side. Repeat this manoeuvre anteriorly for the upper lobes.

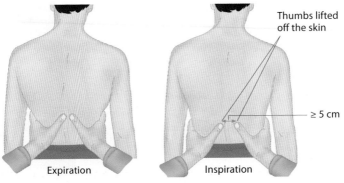

Thumbs lifted
off the skin

≥ 5 cm

Expiration   Inspiration

Figure 5.5 Testing chest expansion for the lower lobes

Vocal fremitus

Palpate the chest wall with the palm of the hand while the patient says 'ninety-nine' aloud. The front and back of the chest are each palpated in two comparable positions with the palm of one hand on each side of the chest. In this way differences in vibration on the chest wall can be detected. This can be a difficult sign to interpret. The causes of change in vocal fremitus are the same as those for vocal resonance (see p. 73).

Ribs

Gently compress the chest wall anteroposteriorly and laterally. Localised pain suggests a rib fracture, which may be secondary to trauma or may be spontaneous as a result of tumour deposition or primary bone disease.

Percussion

With the left hand on the chest wall and the fingers slightly separated and aligned with the ribs, the middle finger is pressed firmly against the chest. Then the pad of the right middle finger is used to strike firmly the middle phalanx of the middle finger of the left hand. The percussing finger is quickly removed so that the note generated is not dampened. The percussing finger must be held partly flexed and a loose swinging movement should come from the wrist and not from the forearm (see Fig 5.6). Percuss on both sides of the anterior, posterior (see Fig 5.7) and axillary regions and in the supraclavicular fossa over the apex of the lung (see Fig 5.8). Percuss the clavicle directly with the percussing finger. For percussion posteriorly, the scapulae can usefully be moved out of the way by asking the patient to move the elbows forward across the front of the chest.

The feel of the percussion note is as important as its sound. The note is affected by the thickness of the chest wall, as well as by underlying structures. Percussion over a solid structure, such as the liver or a consolidated area of lung, produces a **dull note**. Percussion over a fluid-filled area, such as a pleural effusion, produces an extremely dull **(stony dull)** note. Percussion over the normal lung produces a **resonant note**, and percussion over hollow structures such as the bowel or a pneumothorax produces a **hyper-resonant note**.

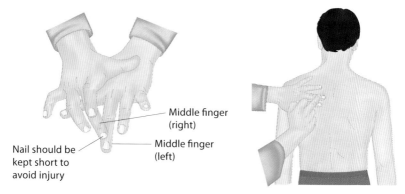

Nail should be kept short to avoid injury

Middle finger (right)

Middle finger (left)

Figure 5.6 Percussion technique

Figure 5.7 Percussing the back

Liver dullness

The upper level of liver dullness is determined by percussing down the anterior chest in the mid-clavicular line. Normally, the upper level of the liver dullness is the fifth rib in the right mid-clavicular line. If the chest is resonant below this level it is a sign of hyperinflation, usually due to emphysema or asthma.

Auscultation

Breath sounds

Using the diaphragm of the stethoscope, listen to the breath sounds in the areas shown in Figure 5.8. Then listen over the back. It is important to compare one side with the other. Remember to listen high up into the axillae and, using the bell of the stethoscope applied above the clavicles, to listen to the lung apices. Listen for the quality and intensity of the breath sounds and for the presence of additional (adventitious) sounds.

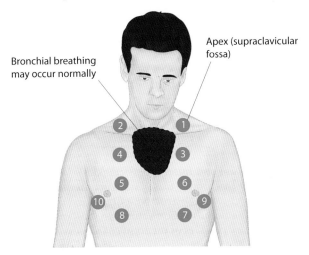

Bronchial breathing may occur normally

Apex (supraclavicular fossa)

Figure 5.8 Where to auscultate

1. *Quality of breath sounds.* Normal breath sounds are heard with the stethoscope over all parts of the chest. They were once thought to arise in the alveoli (vesicles) of the lungs and are therefore called *vesicular sounds.* **Normal (vesicular) breath sounds** are *louder* and *longer* on *inspiration* than on expiration and there is no gap between the inspiratory and expiratory sounds (see Fig 5.9).

   With **bronchial breath sounds**, turbulence in the large airways is heard without being filtered by the alveoli, producing a different sound. Bronchial breath sounds have a hollow, blowing quality. They are audible throughout expiration and there is often a gap between inspiration and expiration. The expiratory sound has a higher intensity and pitch than the inspiratory sound. They are heard over areas of consolidation since solid lung conducts the sound of turbulence in main airways to peripheral areas without filtering.

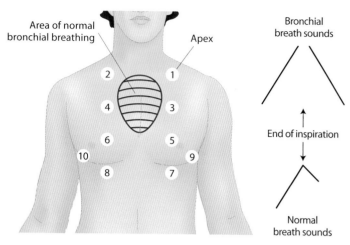

Figure 5.9 Vesicular (normal) and bronchial breath sounds

2. *Intensity of breath sounds.* It is better to describe breath sounds as being of normal or reduced intensity than to speak about air entry. Causes of reduced breath sounds include chronic obstructive pulmonary disease, pleural effusion, pneumothorax, pneumonia, a large neoplasm and pulmonary collapse.

3. *Added (adventitious) sounds.* There are two types of added sounds: continuous (wheezes) and interrupted (crackles). **Wheezes** are usually the result of acute or chronic airway obstruction due to asthma (often high-pitched) or chronic obstructive pulmonary disease (often low-pitched). Interrupted non-musical sounds are best called **crackles**.
   - **Early inspiratory crackles of medium coarseness** are characteristic of chronic obstructive pulmonary disease. They differ from those heard in left ventricular failure, which occur later in the respiratory cycle.
   - **Late or pan-inspiratory crackles** suggest disease confined to the alveoli. They may be fine, medium or coarse in quality:
     - **Fine crackles** have been likened to the sound of hair rubbed between the fingers or to the sound Velcro makes when being unstrapped. They are typically caused by pulmonary fibrosis.
     - **Medium crackles** are often due to left ventricular failure. They can also be present in patients with chronic obstructive pulmonary disease.
     - **Coarse crackles** are characteristic of pools of retained secretions (e.g. bronchiectasis) and have an unpleasant gurgling quality.

4. *Pleural friction rub.* This occurs when thickened, roughened pleural surfaces rub together as the lungs expand and contract; a continuous or intermittent grating sound may be audible. A pleural rub indicates pleurisy, which may be secondary to pulmonary infarction or pneumonia.

If a very localised abnormality is found on auscultation, try to determine the segments involved (see Fig 5.2).

Vocal resonance

Auscultation over the chest while the patient speaks gives further information about the lungs' ability to transmit sounds. Over normal lung the low-pitched components of speech are heard with a booming quality and high-pitched components are attenuated. Ask the patient to say 'ninety-nine' while you listen over each part of the chest. Over consolidated lung the numbers will become clearly audible, whereas over normal lung the sound is muffled. If vocal resonance is present, bronchial breathing is likely to be heard.

The heart

Lay the patient at 45° and examine the jugular venous pressure for evidence of right heart failure. Next examine the praecordium with close attention to the pulmonary component of the second heart sound (P2). This is best heard at the second intercostal space on the left. It should not be louder than the aortic component, best heard at the right second intercostal space. If the P2 is louder, pulmonary hypertension should be strongly suspected.

The peripheral signs of lung disease
The hands
Clubbing

Look for clubbing (see Table 3.2 and Fig 3.3). Respiratory causes of clubbing include carcinoma of the lung and chronic lung suppuration (e.g. pulmonary abscess, tuberculosis). Chronic obstructive pulmonary disease alone does *not* cause clubbing.

Staining from cigarettes

Look for staining of the fingers (actually caused by tar, because nicotine is colourless), a sign of cigarette smoking but not an indication of the number of cigarettes smoked.

Wasting and weakness

Compression and infiltration by a peripheral lung tumour of a lower trunk of the brachial plexus results in wasting of the small muscles of the hands and weakness of finger abduction.

Pulse rate and blood pressure

Tachycardia and pulsus paradoxus (p. 29) are important signs of severe asthma.

Dyspnoea

Watch the patient for signs of dyspnoea at rest. Count the respiratory rate. Tachypnoea (> 25 breaths per minute) means a rapid respiratory rate. Look to see whether the accessory muscles of respiration (the sternomastoids, the platysma and the strap muscles of the neck) are being used (see Fig 5.3).

Character of the cough

Ask the patient to cough several times.
- Lack of the usual explosive beginning may indicate vocal cord paralysis (the 'bovine' cough).
- A muffled, wheezy ineffective cough suggests chronic obstructive pulmonary disease.
- A very loose, productive cough suggests excessive bronchial secretions due to chronic bronchitis, pneumonia or bronchiectasis.
- A dry, irritating cough may occur with chest infection, asthma or carcinoma of the bronchus and less commonly with left ventricular failure or interstitial lung disease.

Sputum

Note the volume and type of sputum (purulent, mucoid or muco-purulent). Record the presence or absence of blood.

Stridor

Obstruction of the larynx, trachea or large airways may cause stridor, a rasping or croaking noise loudest on inspiration. This can be due to a foreign body, a tumour, an infection (e.g. epiglottitis) or inflammation.

Hoarseness

Listen to the voice for hoarseness. Causes can include laryngitis, vocal cord tumour, recurrent laryngeal nerve palsy (e.g. from an apical lung cancer) or gastro-oesophageal reflux.

The eyes and tongue

A constricted pupil and a partial ptosis (partial closure of one eyelid) comprise **Horner's syndrome** (p. 147). This can be due to an apical lung tumour compressing the sympathetic nerves in the neck.

Look for central **cyanosis** by inspecting the tongue.

The trachea

Standing in front of the patient, push the forefinger of the right hand very gently up and backwards from the suprasternal notch until the trachea is felt. If the trachea is displaced to one side, its edge rather than its middle will be felt and a larger space will be present on one side than the other (see Fig 5.10). Slight displacement to the right is fairly common in healthy people. This examination is uncomfortable for the patient so be gentle.

Significant displacement of the trachea suggests, but is not specific for, disease of the *upper lobes of the lung*.

Feel for a *tracheal tug*—the finger resting on the trachea feels it move inferiorly with each inspiration. This is a sign of gross overexpansion of the chest because of airflow obstruction.

Perform the *forced expiratory time test*. Ask the patient to take in a maximum inspiration, then exhale forcibly and completely through the open mouth. Normal is 3 seconds or less. A forced expiratory time of 9 seconds or more is strongly suggestive of chronic obstructive pulmonary disease.

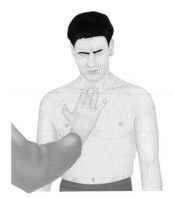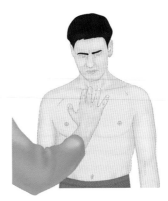

Figure 5.10 Feeling for the position of the trachea

The chest OSCE: hints panel

1   This woman has a problem with cough. Take a history from her.

   (a) Ask her about the cough: how long, whether it is productive or not, is getting better or worse, is worse lying down and prevents sleep.

   (b) Ask about the sputum: volume, colour etc.

   (c) Ask about dyspnoea, wheeze and pleuritic chest pain.

   (d) Ask her about any history of known lung disease, including the details.

   (e) Ask her about any current medications.

   (f) Synthesise and present your findings.

2   This man has been breathless. Take an occupational history from him.

   (a) Ask him the following:

      (i)   What is your job?

      (ii) What does this involve, in detail? How long have you been doing this work?

      (iii) What ventilation arrangements are provided at work?

      (iv) Are you or other workers or customers permitted to smoke at work?

      (v)   Does your work involve exposure to dusts, solvents or animals? (If this is not already clear.)

      (vi) What previous work have you done? What did that involve?

      (vii) Have you any hobbies or pets?

   (b) Present your findings and outline the possible risk associated with any exposure.

3   This man has chest pain made worse by inspiration and breathlessness. Please examine him.

   (a) If necessary, ask the patient to undress to the waist. Look for wasting and pallor, nail clubbing and cigarette staining of the fingers, and pain on inspiration (pleuritic chest pain).

   (b) Record his respiratory rate and take his temperature.

   (c) Sit him over the side of the bed or ask him to sit upright.

(d) Stand back and look for central cyanosis (tongue), bruising (trauma) and red raised skin lesions (vasculitis).

(e) Feel the trachea position. Is it mid-line?

(f) Examine the chest first from the front and then from the back: inspect, palpate, percuss and auscultate. Note any signs of a friction rub, pneumonia or a pleural effusion.

(g) Lay the patient at 45° and assess his pulse, blood pressure, JVP and praecordium (pulmonary embolus).

(h) Assess his lower legs for pitting oedema (bilateral) and signs of deep venous thrombosis (unilateral).

(i) Synthesise and present your findings.

4 **This man has haemoptysis and weight loss. Please examine him.**

(a) Look for obvious evidence of weight loss or cachexia.

(b) Carefully inspect the nails of his hands for clubbing and look for wrist swelling (hypertrophic osteoarthropathy).

(c) Feel for cervical and other lymph node groups.

(d) Examine his chest systematically. Particularly look for unilateral signs that might indicate a lung cancer (e.g. evidence of mediastinal shift, local area of dullness, signs of an effusion).

The chest history and examination
hints for success

1 Dyspnoea of respiratory cause can sometimes be difficult to distinguish from cardiac dyspnoea, but a careful history can be diagnostic.

2 The smoking history and occupational history are particularly important in any patient with respiratory symptoms.

3 Production of sputum and particularly the presence of haemoptysis must be documented. Available sputum should be inspected.

4 Inspect for chest wall symmetry, palpate for expansion, percuss for dullness and auscultate for abnormal or reduced breath sounds. Examination of the upper lobes should not be forgotten.

5 Although a systematic and complete examination is essential, you may elect to examine the posterior chest (lower lobes) first, since in most cases 'this is where the money is' in respiratory disease.

6 Chronic obstructive pulmonary disease is suggested by a history of smoking, the presence of wheeze, early inspiratory crackles and diminished breath sounds.

7 Absence of clinical signs does not exclude a respiratory disease; the clinical signs can be less sensitive than investigations such as a chest X-ray (e.g. for detection of a mass lesion) or spirometry (e.g. airflow limitation).

chapter 6

The abdomen

Gut: The long pipe stretching with many convolutions from the stomach to the vent.

S Johnson, *A Dictionary Of The English Language* (1755)

This chapter presents an introduction to history taking and examination of conditions whose signs are found chiefly in the abdomen. Gastrointestinal, haematological and renal disease can present with abdominal symptoms and signs, and these are all discussed in this chapter.

The gastrointestinal history

When the history suggests a probable gastrointestinal problem, the examination is directed at the gastrointestinal system and begins with the peripheral signs of gut disease, as set out below.

The gastrointestinal system assessment sequence

1 Presenting symptoms, e.g. abdominal pain, loss of weight or appetite, difficulty swallowing, nausea and vomiting, diarrhoea or constipation, rectal bleeding, jaundice
2 Detailed questions about presenting symptoms (SOCRATES, p. 4)
3 Questions about previous gastrointestinal problems, procedures or operations and risk factors, e.g. viral hepatitis, excess alcohol consumption
4 Examination for peripheral signs of gastrointestinal disease
5 Examination of the abdomen: areas of tenderness, liver and spleen, other masses, ascites, bowel sounds etc
6 Rectal examination
7 Provisional and differential diagnosis

Presenting symptoms (see Table 6.1)

Table 6.1 The gastrointestinal history: presenting symptoms
Major symptoms
Abdominal pain
Appetite and/or weight change
Nausea and/or vomiting
Heartburn and/or acid regurgitation
Waterbrash
Dysphagia
Disturbed defecation (diarrhoea, constipation, faecal incontinence)
Bleeding (haematemesis, melaena, rectal bleeding)
Jaundice
Dark urine, pale stools
Abdominal swelling
Pruritus
Lethargy
Fever

Abdominal pain

Careful history taking will often lead to the correct diagnosis of the cause of abdominal pain. As usual, the following aspects should be considered: **frequency** and **duration**, **severity**, **site** and **radiation**, **character** and **pattern**, **exacerbating** and **relieving factors**, and **associated symptoms (e.g. fever)**.

Frequency and duration

Find out when the pain began, how often attacks have occurred and how long they last. Abdominal pain may be acute or chronic.

Severity

Grade the pain from 0 to 10. Also find out how much the pain interferes with normal activities. A four-point grading (mild, moderate, severe, very severe) is an alternative.

Site and radiation

Ask the patient to point to the area affected and the site of maximum intensity. Ask whether the pain travels elsewhere. Pain due to pancreatic disease or a penetrating peptic ulcer (now rare) often radiates through to the back. Pain may radiate to the shoulder with diaphragmatic irritation or to the neck with oesophageal reflux.

Character and pattern

Colicky pain comes and goes in waves and is related to peristaltic movements; it suggests bowel or ureteric obstruction. Pain from biliary tract disease is not usually colicky but constant and severe. If the pain is **chronic**, ask whether there is a daily pattern of pain.

6

Exacerbating and relieving factors

Pain due to peptic ulceration may be related to meals. Eating may precipitate ischaemic pain in the small bowel (mesenteric angina) and lead to weight loss. Antacids or vomiting may relieve peptic ulcer pain or that of gastro-oesophageal reflux. Defecation or passage of flatus may temporarily relieve the pain of any colonic disease. Patients who obtain some relief by rolling around vigorously are more likely to have a colicky pain, whereas those who lie perfectly still are more likely to have peritonitis.

Patterns of pain

Peptic ulcer disease

This is classically a dull or burning pain in the epigastrium (see Fig 6.1) that is relieved by food or antacids and may occur postprandially. It is typically episodic and may occur at night, waking the patient from sleep. It is not possible to distinguish duodenal ulceration from gastric ulceration clinically. The most common cause of epigastric pain is functional (non-ulcer) dyspepsia, not peptic ulceration.

Pancreatic pain

This is often a steady, epigastric pain or ache that may be partly relieved by sitting up and leaning forward. There is often radiation of the pain to the back.

Biliary pain

Although usually called 'biliary colic' this is rarely colicky; it is usually a severe, constant, right upper quadrant or epigastric pain that can last for hours and occurs episodically and irregularly. Cystic duct obstruction often causes epigastric pain. If cholecystitis develops, the pain typically shifts to the right upper quadrant and becomes more severe. The pain may also radiate across the upper abdomen and around to the right side of the back in the scapular region.

Renal colic

This is very severe colicky pain superimposed on a background of constant pain in the renal angle, often radiating towards the groin.

Bowel obstruction

Peri-umbilical pain suggests a small bowel origin but colonic pain can occur anywhere in the abdomen. Small bowel obstruction tends to cause more frequent colicky pain (with a cycle every 2–3 minutes) than large bowel obstruction (every 10–15 minutes). Bowel obstruction is often associated with vomiting, constipation (failure to pass flatus or stool) and abdominal distension.

Functional bowel disease (irritable bowel syndrome)

Pain for which no structural cause can be found is common among patients with gastrointestinal symptoms. Irritable bowel syndrome (IBS) is associated with bloating and disturbed bowel habit (constipation, diarrhoea or alternating symptoms). The pain is typically relieved by defecation. Its course can be very prolonged but tends to be intermittent, and it may wax and wane over many years.

Appetite or weight change

The presence of both anorexia (loss of appetite) and weight loss should make one suspicious of an underlying malignancy, but they may also occur with depression. The combination of weight loss with an increased appetite suggests malabsorption of nutrients or a hypermetabolic state (e.g. thyrotoxicosis).

Nausea and vomiting

Nausea is the sensation of wanting to vomit. There are many gastrointestinal causes (e.g. peptic ulceration or gastric cancer causing pyloric outlet obstruction) and non-gastrointestinal causes (e.g. labyrinthitis, many drugs, migraine, brain stem tumour, renal failure) of nausea and vomiting. The volume and nature of the vomitus may suggest the cause of the problem. Vomiting of large volumes, but infrequently, suggests gastric outlet obstruction; the frequent vomiting of bile or faecal material suggests bowel obstruction.

Heartburn and acid regurgitation

Heartburn refers to the presence of a burning pain or discomfort in the retrosternal area due to reflux of acid from the stomach into the oesophagus. Typically, this sensation travels up towards the throat and occurs after meals, or is aggravated by bending, stooping or lying supine. Antacids usually relieve the pain, at least transiently. **Acid regurgitation** is an acid (sour) taste in the mouth that is due to reflux. **Waterbrash** refers to tasteless liquid (saliva) filling the mouth; this can occur in patients with peptic ulceration, but is not usually a symptom of oesophageal reflux. Extra-oesophageal manifestations of gastro-oesophageal reflux disease (GORD) can include **chest pain**, chronic **cough**, symptoms of **asthma**, and **hoarseness**.

Dysphagia

Dysphagia is difficulty swallowing. Such difficulty may occur with solids or liquids. If a patient complains of difficulty swallowing, it is important to differentiate painful swallowing from actual difficulty. Painful swallowing is termed **odynophagia** and occurs with any severe inflammatory process involving the oesophagus.

If the patient complains of difficulty initiating swallowing or complains of fluid regurgitating into the nose or choking on trying to swallow, this suggests that the cause of the dysphagia is in the pharynx (**pharyngeal dysphagia**).

If the patient complains of food sticking after swallowing, it is important to consider causes of oesophageal blockage (e.g. carcinoma or stricture). If these patients also have symptoms of reflux, this suggests a stricture caused by oesophagitis. If there has been significant weight loss, this suggests cancer. A history of **intermittent food impaction** suggests eosinophilic oesophagitis.

Diarrhoea

Diarrhoea can be defined in a number of ways. Patients may complain of frequent stools (more than three per day being abnormal) or they may complain of a change in the consistency of the stools, which have become loose or watery.

When a history of diarrhoea is obtained, it is also important to determine whether this has occurred acutely or is a chronic problem. Acute diarrhoea is more likely to be infectious in nature, while chronic diarrhoea has a large number of causes.

Consider, in chronic cases:

1. *Secretory diarrhoea.* The stools are of large volume (often more than 1 L a day) and the diarrhoea persists when the patient is fasting. Secretory diarrhoea may be caused by a villous adenoma or, rarely, a tumour which secretes vasoactive intestinal peptide (VIP).
2. *Osmotic diarrhoea.* The diarrhoea disappears when the patient fasts (e.g. due to lactose intolerance, malabsorption or the taking of a non-absorbed osmotic laxative).
3. *Exudative diarrhoea.* The stools are of small volume but frequent and there is associated blood or mucus (e.g. colon cancer or inflammatory bowel disease).
4. *Malabsorption.* If there is steatorrhoea (excess fat in the stools), the stools are pale, foul smelling and difficult to flush away (e.g. chronic pancreatitis, coeliac sprue).
5. *Increased intestinal motility* (e.g. thyrotoxicosis). Here the stools may be normal in consistency and an increased bowel frequency may not be volunteered as a symptom.

Constipation

It is important to determine what patients mean if they say they are constipated. Constipation is a common symptom and can refer to the passage of infrequent stools (fewer than three times per week is abnormal), hard stools or stools that are difficult to evacuate (i.e. require excessive straining). This symptom may occur acutely or it may be a chronic problem. Chronic causes include colonic obstruction (e.g. cancer), metabolic disease (e.g. hypothyroidism, diabetes) or rectal outlet blockage (e.g. from a failure to relax the external anal sphincter on straining).

Mucus

The passage of mucus (white flecks on the stool) may occur in inflammatory bowel disease or the irritable bowel syndrome or with rectal carcinomas or villous adenomas.

Bleeding

Patients may present with haematemesis (vomiting blood), melaena (passage of jet-black stools) or haematochezia (passage of bright-red blood per rectum). Bright red blood on the outside of the stool suggests outlet bleeding (e.g. from haemorrhoids), whereas blood mixed in the stool suggests colonic disease. With occult bleeding from the bowel, patients may present with symptoms and signs of anaemia (e.g. fatigue and pallor).

Jaundice

Usually the patient's relatives notice a yellow discolouration of the sclera or skin due to bilirubin deposition before the patient does. A careful history and examination will reveal the correct diagnosis of the cause of jaundice in two-thirds of patients. Ask about other symptoms, including:

1. abdominal pain: gallstones, for example, can cause biliary pain and jaundice
2. change in the colour of the stools and urine: obstructive jaundice (e.g. blockage of the common bile duct by a gallstone or carcinoma of the pancreas) causes dark urine and pale stools, whereas haemolytic anaemia is associated with dark urine and normal-coloured stools
3. fever and malaise (e.g. viral hepatitis or drug reactions).

Past history

Ask about:

1. surgical procedures, blood transfusions and anaesthetics
2. relapsing and remitting pain in the past (suggesting peptic ulceration) in a patient with sudden severe pain (perforated peptic ulcer)
3. a diagnosis of inflammatory bowel disease and any treatment received
4. use of non-steroidal anti-inflammatory drugs (NSAIDs).

Social history

Ask about:

1. the patient's occupation
2. recent travel (e.g. to countries where hepatitis is endemic)
3. alcohol intake
4. contact with people who have been jaundiced
5. use of intravenous drugs.

Family history

A family history of colon or gastric cancer, inflammatory bowel disease or liver disease is often relevant.

The genitourinary history

The genitourinary system assessment also involves a careful abdominal examination. The sequence is set out below.

The genitourinary system assessment sequence

1 Presenting symptoms, e.g. changes in the urine or symptoms during micturition (pain, poor stream nocturia), abdominal or flank pain, fever, malaise
2 Detailed questions about presenting symptoms (SOCRATES, p. 4)
3 Questions about previous urinary problems and procedures or operations, known abnormalities of kidney function, risk factors for kidney disease (e.g. hypertension, diabetes mellitus)
4 History of dialysis or renal transplantation
5 Blood pressure, and examination for peripheral signs of renal failure or dialysis
6 Examination of the abdomen: renal masses, peritoneal dialysis fluid
7 Examination of the genitals, if appropriate, and of the urine
8 Provisional and differential diagnosis

Presenting symptoms (see Table 6.2)

Table 6.2 The genitourinary history: presenting symptoms

Major symptoms

Change in appearance of urine (e.g. haematuria—red discolouration)

Change in urine volume or stream

  Polyuria (an increase in the volume of urine)

  Nocturia (getting up to pass urine during the night)

  Oliguria (reduced urine output: < 400 mL/day)

  Anuria (little or no urine output: < 50 mL/day)

  Symptoms of prostatic enlargement

    Decrease in stream size

    Hesitancy

    Dribbling

    Urine retention

    Urinary frequency

    Urinary urgency (the need to pass urine without delay)

Incontinence of urine (stress incontinence, e.g. on coughing; urge incontinence)

Double voiding (incomplete bladder emptying)

Renal colic

Symptoms of urinary infection

  Dysuria (painful micturition), frequency (the need to pass small amounts of urine frequently), urgency, fever, loin pain

Urethral discharge

Symptoms suggestive of chronic renal failure (uraemia)

  Oliguria, nocturia, polyuria

  Anorexia, a metallic taste, vomiting, fatigue, hiccups, insomnia

  Itch, bruising, oedema

Erectile dysfunction

Loss of libido

Infertility

Urethral or vaginal discharge

Genital rash

Patients may present with urinary tract symptoms (changes in the urine or in micturition) or abdominal or flank pain. Many patients have no symptoms but are found to be hypertensive or to have abnormalities on routine urinalysis or serum biochemistry.

Ask about a change in the appearance of the urine, symptoms of urinary obstruction (e.g. hesitancy, decrease in the size of the stream, terminal dribbling) and urinary incontinence. Ask about symptoms of renal failure: these are not specific but can include nocturia, anorexia, vomiting, fatigue, hiccups, insomnia and pruritus.

A **menstrual history** should always be obtained (including the date of menarche and the regularity of the menstrual cycle). Ask about dysmenorrhoea (painful menstruation), menorrhagia (abnormally heavy periods), vaginal discharge, the number of pregnancies and births, complications of pregnancy and childbirth (e.g. hypertension), and contraceptive methods.

Past history

Find out about recurrent urinary tract infections or calculi, renal surgery, any previous detection of proteinuria or microscopic haematuria, a diagnosis of diabetes mellitus, gout or hypertension, or the performance of a renal biopsy.

Social history

Ask about any social problems, and in renal failure patients ask how the patient has coped and is coping with a serious chronic illness.

Treatment

A detailed drug history must be taken. Find out whether the patient is undergoing dialysis and whether this is haemodialysis or peritoneal dialysis.

A common form of treatment for renal failure is renal transplantation. A patient may be well informed about graft function, rejection episodes and drug treatment.

Family history

Ask particularly about polycystic kidney disease, diabetes mellitus and hypertension in the family.

The haematological history

The haematological examination begins with a search for peripheral signs and extends to an abdominal examination. The sequence is set out below.

The haematological system assessment sequence

1   Presenting symptoms, e.g. lethargy, dyspnoea, pallor, easy bruising, abdominal pain, lymph node enlargement
2   Detailed questions about presenting symptoms (SOCRATES, p. 4)
3   Questions about previous haematological problems and procedures, known blood test results
4   Examination for peripheral signs of haematological disease including all lymph node groups
5   Examination of the abdomen: hepatosplenomegaly
6   Provisional and differential diagnosis

Presenting symptoms (see Table 6.3)

Patients may present with symptoms of anaemia (e.g. lethargy, palpitations, dyspnoea on exertion or angina). Alternatively, the presenting symptoms may be of the condition leading to anaemia or of the causes of anaemia (e.g. rectal bleeding or the bowel symptoms of malabsorption). The patient

Table 6.3 The haematological history: presenting symptoms

Major symptoms

Symptoms of anaemia: weakness, tiredness, dyspnoea, fatigue, postural dizziness

Bleeding (menstrual, gastrointestinal)

Easy bruising

Thrombotic tendency (e.g. repeated deep venous thrombosis in the legs)

Infection, fever

Jaundice

Lymph gland enlargement

Bone pain

Paraesthesiae (e.g. vitamin B_{12} deficiency)

Skin rash

Weight loss

Night sweats

who complains of lymph node enlargement should be asked about night sweats and weight loss (e.g. lymphoma). Recurrent infection with fevers may be the first symptom of a disorder of the immune system or of neutropenia. Take a detailed history from patients who easily bruise or bleed, including questions about postoperative bleeding. If bleeding after trauma is immediate, this suggests a platelet problem; if bleeding occurs after a delay, a clotting factor problem is more likely.

Past history

Ask about systemic disease and previous gastric surgery as causes of anaemia. Ask whether the patient has been refused as a blood donor and, if so, why.

Treatment

Find out about iron supplements or vitamin B_{12} injections, and the use of NSAIDs, anticoagulants or chemotherapy. Find out whether previous blood transfusions or venesections have been required.

Family history

There may be a family history of thalassaemia, haemolytic anaemia (or jaundice), haemophilia, von Willebrand's disease or factor V Leiden deficiency.

Examination anatomy

A knowledge of the underlying structures of the abdomen helps explain the various examination techniques. As with the chest examination, try to picture the structures that lie beneath the surface of the area being examined (see Fig 6.1).

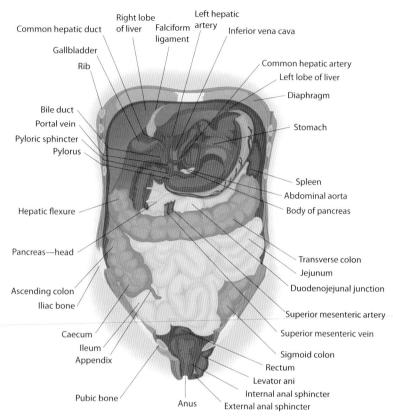

Figure 6.1 The abdominal organs

Examining the abdomen

The abdomen should be examined by **inspection**, **palpation**, **percussion** and **auscultation**.

Inspection

The patient should **lie flat** (see Fig 6.2), with one pillow under the head and with the abdomen exposed from the nipples to the pubic symphysis. Inspection begins with a careful look for abdominal **scars**, which may indicate previous surgery or trauma. Look in the area around the umbilicus for small laparoscopic surgical scars. Older scars are white whereas recent scars are pink because the tissue remains vascular. Note the presence of **stomas** (colostomy, ileostomy or ileal conduit), fistulae or a peritoneal dialysis catheter. Nephrectomy scars are often more posterior than might be expected; they usually lie in the flank as far posterior as the erector spinae muscle group. Renal transplant scars are usually found in the right or left lower abdomen (iliac fossae). A **transplanted kidney** may be visible

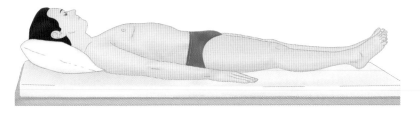

Figure 6.2 Abdominal examination: positioning the patient

as a bulge under the scar. Previous peritoneal dialysis results in small scars from catheter placement in the peritoneal cavity; these are situated on the lower abdomen at or near the mid-line.

Generalised abdominal **distension** may be present. All the causes of this sound as though they begin with the letter 'F': fat (gross obesity), fluid (ascites), fetus, flatus (gaseous distension due to bowel obstruction), faeces, filthy big tumour (e.g. large polycystic kidneys or an ovarian tumour) or phantom pregnancy (looks pregnant but isn't). When the peritoneal cavity is filled with large volumes of fluid (ascites) from whatever cause, the abdominal flanks and wall appear tense and the umbilicus is shallow or everted and points downwards.

Local swellings may indicate enlargement of one of the abdominal or pelvic organs or weakening of the abdominal wall as a result of previous surgery (**incisional hernia**).

Prominent **veins** may be obvious on the abdominal wall in patients with severe portal hypertension or inferior vena cava obstruction.

Pulsations may be visible. An expanding central pulsation in the epigastrium suggests an abdominal aortic aneurysm. However, the abdominal aorta can often be seen to pulsate in normal thin people.

Visible peristalsis usually suggests intestinal obstruction.

Skin lesions should also be noted. These include the vesicles of herpes zoster, which occur in a radicular pattern (they are localised to only one side of the abdomen in the distribution of a single nerve root). Herpes zoster may be responsible for severe abdominal pain that is of mysterious origin until the rash appears. Skin tattoos may indicate an increased risk of hepatitis B or C infection.

Stretching of the abdominal wall severe enough to cause rupture of the elastic fibres in the skin produces pink linear marks with a wrinkled appearance, which are called **striae**. When these are wide and purple-coloured, Cushing's syndrome (from steroid hormone excess) may be the cause. Ascites and pregnancy are much more common causes of striae.

Next, squat down beside the bed so that the patient's abdomen is at eye level. Ask the patient to take slow deep breaths through the mouth and watch for the movement of a large liver in the right upper quadrant (see below) or spleen in the left upper quadrant. Ask the patient to cough and look for the reducible swellings that indicate hernias. These may be present under scars (incisional hernias) or in the inguinal region.

Palpation

Reassure the patient that the examination will not be painful and use warm hands. Ask whether any particular area is tender and examine this area last.

For descriptive purposes the abdomen has been divided into **nine regions**, or **four quadrants** (see Fig 6.3(a) and (b)). Palpation in each region is performed with the palmar surface of the fingers acting together. For the palpation of the edges of organs or masses, the lateral surface of the forefinger is the most sensitive part of the hand.

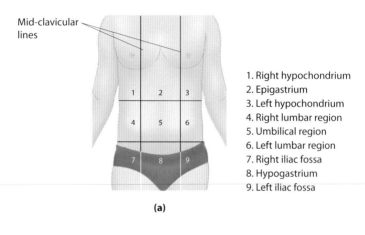

Mid-clavicular lines

1. Right hypochondrium
2. Epigastrium
3. Left hypochondrium
4. Right lumbar region
5. Umbilical region
6. Left lumbar region
7. Right iliac fossa
8. Hypogastrium
9. Left iliac fossa

(a)

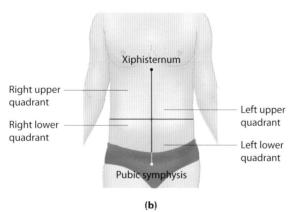

Xiphisternum

Right upper quadrant

Right lower quadrant

Left upper quadrant

Left lower quadrant

Pubic symphysis

(b)

Figure 6.3 (a) Regions of the abdomen **(b)** Quadrants of the abdomen

Palpation should begin with **light pressure** in each region. Stop straight away if this causes pain for the patient. All the movements of the hand should occur at the metacarpophalangeal joints and the hand should be moulded to the shape of the abdominal wall. Note the presence of any tenderness or masses in each region.

Deep palpation of the abdomen is performed next. Deep palpation is used to detect deeper masses and to define those already discovered. Ask the patient about tenderness. Any mass must be characterised and described (see box below).

Descriptive features of intra-abdominal masses

For any abdominal mass *all* the following should be determined:

1 site: the region involved and depth (abdominal wall or intra-abdominal)
2 size (which should be measured) and shape
3 tenderness
4 surface, which may be regular or irregular
5 edge, which may be regular or irregular
6 consistency, which may be hard or soft
7 mobility and movement with inspiration
8 whether it is pulsatile or not
9 whether one can get above the mass.

Guarding of the abdomen, when resistance to palpation occurs due to contraction of the abdominal muscles, may result from tenderness or anxiety, and may be voluntary or **involuntary**. The latter suggests peritonitis. **Rigidity** is a constant involuntary contraction of the abdominal muscles always associated with tenderness and indicates peritoneal irritation. **Rebound tenderness** is said to be present when the abdominal wall, having been compressed slowly, is released rapidly and a sudden stab of pain results. This may make the patient wince so the patient's face should be watched while this manoeuvre is performed. It strongly suggests the presence of peritonitis. If the abdomen is very tender, light percussion will give the same information and cause less discomfort.

The liver

Feel for hepatomegaly (see Fig 6.4). With the examining hand aligned parallel to the right costal margin, and beginning in the right iliac fossa, ask the patient to breathe in and out slowly through the mouth. With each expiration the hand is advanced by 1 or 2 cm closer to the right costal margin. During inspiration the hand is kept still and the lateral margin of the forefinger waits expectantly for the liver edge to strike it.

If the liver is palpable, its surface should be felt. The edge of the liver and the surface itself may be:

1. hard or soft
2. tender or non-tender
3. regular or irregular
4. pulsatile or non-pulsatile.

The normal liver edge may be palpable just below the right costal margin on deep inspiration, especially in thin people. The edge is then felt to be soft and regular with a fairly sharply defined border, and the surface of the liver itself is smooth.

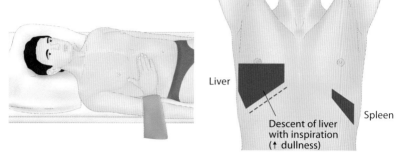

Figure 6.4 Abdominal examination: the liver

If the liver edge is palpable, the total **liver span** should be measured. The normal upper border of the liver is level with the fifth rib in the mid-clavicular line. At this point the percussion note over the chest changes from resonant to dull (p. 92). To estimate the liver span, percuss down along the right mid-clavicular line until the liver dullness is encountered and measure from here to the palpable liver edge. The normal span is less than 13 cm.

The gall bladder

The gall bladder is occasionally palpable below the right costal margin where this crosses the lateral border of the rectus muscles, but this does not occur in health. If biliary obstruction or gall bladder disease is suspected, the examining hand should be oriented perpendicular to the costal margin, feeling from medial to lateral. Unlike the liver edge, the gall bladder, if palpable, will be a bulbous, focal rounded mass that moves downwards on inspiration.

Murphy's sign should be sought if cholecystitis is suspected. While taking a deep breath in, the patient catches his or her breath when an inflamed gall bladder presses on the examiner's hand, which is lying at the costal margin.

The spleen

The spleen enlarges inferiorly and medially. Its edge should be sought below the umbilicus in the mid-line initially. A **two-handed technique** is recommended. The left hand is placed posterolaterally just below the left lower ribs and the right hand is placed on the abdomen parallel to the left costal margin. Don't start palpation too near the costal margin or a large spleen will be missed. As the right hand is advanced closer to the left costal margin, the left hand compresses firmly over the rib cage so as to produce a loose fold of skin; this removes tension from the abdominal wall and enables a slightly enlarged soft spleen to be felt as it moves down towards the right iliac fossa at the end of inspiration.

If the spleen is not palpable, roll the patient onto the right side towards you and repeat the palpation (see Fig 6.5), beginning close to the left costal margin.

6

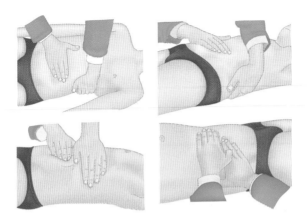

Figure 6.5 Palpation of the spleen
(a) Palpation begins in the lower mid-abdomen and finishes up under the left costal margin.
(b) Your hand supports the patient's side …
(c) … and then rests over the lower costal margin to reduce skin resistance.
(d) If the spleen is not palpable when the patient is flat, the patient should be rolled towards you and two-handed palpation is repeated.

The kidneys

An attempt to palpate both the kidneys should be a routine part of the examination. Use a **bimanual method**. Lie the patient flat on his or her back. To palpate the right kidney, slide the hand underneath the patient's back to rest with the heel of the hand under the right loin. The fingers remain free to flex at the metacarpophalangeal joints in the area of the renal angle. The flexing fingers can push the contents of the abdomen anteriorly. The other hand is placed over the right upper quadrant (see Fig 6.6).

When ballotting the kidneys, the renal angle is pressed sharply by the flexing fingers of the posterior hand. The kidney can be felt to float upwards and strike the anterior hand. Then try to palpate the left kidney. The lower

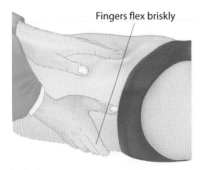

Fingers flex briskly

Figure 6.6 Ballotting the kidneys

pole of the right kidney may be palpable in normal thin people. Both kidneys move downwards only a little with inspiration.

It is particularly common to **confuse a large left kidney with an enlarged spleen**. The major distinguishing features are:

1. The spleen has no palpable upper border—you cannot feel the space between the spleen and the costal margin, which is present in renal enlargement.
2. The spleen, unlike the kidney, has a notch anteromedially, which may be palpable.
3. The spleen moves inferomedially on inspiration, whereas the kidney moves inferiorly.
4. The spleen is not usually ballottable unless gross ascites is present, but the kidney is, again because of its retroperitoneal position.
5. The percussion note is dull over the spleen but is usually resonant over the kidney, because the latter lies posterior to loops of gas-filled bowel.
6. A friction rub may occasionally be heard over the spleen, but never over the kidney, because it is too posterior.

Percussion

Percussion is used to define the size and nature of organs and masses, and to detect fluid in the peritoneal cavity. It is reliable for the detection of an enlarged liver and may be more sensitive than palpation for detecting a mildly enlarged spleen. Percuss over the lowest intercostal space in the left anterior axillary line, in both inspiration and expiration, with the patient supine. Splenomegaly should be suspected if the percussion note is dull or becomes dull on complete inspiration.

Ascites

Begin with percussion starting in the mid-line with the finger pointing towards the feet; the percussion note is tested out towards the flanks on each side (see Fig 6.7).

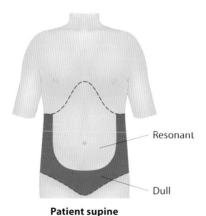

Resonant

Dull

Patient supine

Figure 6.7 Testing for shifting dullness

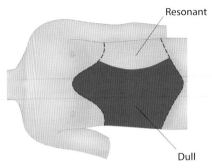

Patient on right side

Figure 6.7 Testing for shifting dullness *continued*

If **dullness in the flanks** is detected, the sign of **shifting dullness** should be sought. Stand on the right side of the bed and percuss out to the left flank until dullness is reached. This point should be marked with a finger or a pen (not an indelible one) and the patient asked to roll towards you. After 30 seconds or so repeat percussion over the marked point. If fluid shifts, the dullness will disappear. Shifting dullness is present if the area of dullness has changed to become resonant.

Auscultation

Listen for bowel sounds, bruits and rubs

Bowel sounds

Place the diaphragm of the stethoscope just below the umbilicus. In normal healthy people bowel sounds can be heard over all parts of the abdomen. They have a soft, gurgling character and occur only intermittently. Bowel sounds should be described as either **present** or **absent**. Complete absence of bowel sounds (over a 3-minute period with the stethoscope in one place) indicates **paralytic ileus**.

An obstructed bowel produces a louder and more high-pitched sound with a **tinkling** quality, which is due to the presence of air and liquid ('obstructed bowel sounds'). Intestinal hurry or rush, which may occur in diarrhoeal states, causes loud gurgling sounds (borborygmi), which are often audible without the stethoscope.

Other sounds

Abdominal bruits (high-pitched, mostly systolic sounds) may be audible over the liver in the presence of hepatocellular cancer. Continuous sound may be caused by arteriovenous shunts related to portal hypertension. Renal bruits (heard on either side of the mid-line above the umbilicus) may indicate renal artery stenosis, but soft abdominal bruits are a common normal finding.

A **friction rub** (creaking or grating noise) may be audible as the patient breathes in and out when the peritoneum is inflamed. This rare sign may be the result of a hepatic or splenic infarct, or of malignant deposits.

The groin

Examine the inguinal lymph nodes, look for hernias and palpate the testes.

Inguinal lymph nodes

There are two groups: one along the inguinal ligament and the other along the femoral vessels. A method of characterising palpable lymph nodes is summarised in the box below. Small (<1 cm diameter), firm mobile nodes are commonly found in healthy people.

Characteristics of lymph nodes

During the palpation of lymph nodes the following features must be considered.

Site

Palpable nodes may be localised to one region (e.g. local infection, early lymphoma) or be generalised (e.g. late lymphoma). The palpable lymph node areas are:

- epitrochlear
- axillary
- cervical (includes occipital and supraclavicular)
- para-aortic (rarely palpable)
- inguinal
- popliteal.

Size

Large nodes are usually abnormal (>1 cm).

Consistency

- Hard nodes suggest carcinoma deposits.
- Soft nodes may be normal.
- Rubbery nodes may be due to lymphoma.

Tenderness

This implies infection or acute inflammation.

Fixation

Nodes that are fixed to underlying structures are more likely to be infiltrated by carcinoma than mobile nodes.

Overlying skin

Inflammation of the overlying skin suggests infection, and tethering to the overlying skin suggests carcinoma.

Hernias

In the patient with an acute abdomen, a strangulated hernia must be excluded as a cause in all cases. If a hernia is not obvious while the patient is lying down, complete examination requires that the patient be examined while standing.

A summary of the relevant surface anatomy is shown in Figure 6.8.

6

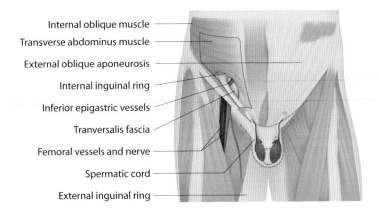

Internal oblique muscle
Transverse abdominus muscle
External oblique aponeurosis
Internal inguinal ring
Inferior epigastric vessels
Tranversalis fascia
Femoral vessels and nerve
Spermatic cord
External inguinal ring

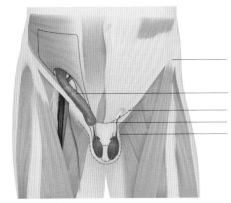

Anterior superior iliac spine

Indirect inguinal hernia
Abdominal crease
Pubic tubercle
Groin crease

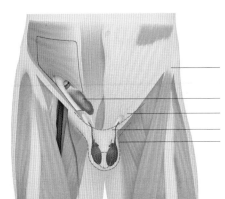

Anterior superior iliac spine

Direct inguinal hernia
Abdominal crease
Pubic tubercle
Groin crease

Figure 6.8 Anatomy of the inguinal region and types of hernias

Inguinal hernias

An **inguinal hernia** typically bulges *above* the crease of the groin. Confirm the position of the swelling in the groin above or below the inguinal ligament, which lies between the anterior superior iliac spine and the pubic tubercle. The pubic tubercle is found just above the attachment of the adductor longus tendon to the pubic bone, which can be felt on the upper medial aspect of the thigh. If the swelling lies *medial to* and *above* the pubic tubercle, it is likely to be an inguinal hernia (see Fig 6.9(a)). The characteristic inguinal hernia is a soft lump that can usually be pushed back into the abdominal cavity (i.e. it is reducible), and an impulse is palpable if the patient coughs. The cough impulse must always be sought. Next examine the scrotum (see below).

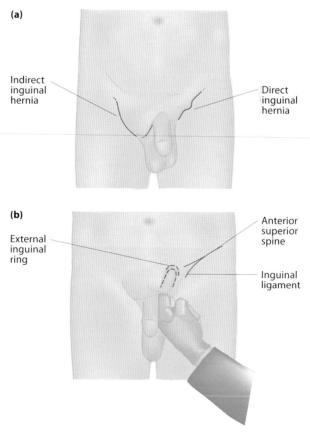

Figure 6.9 (a) Note the elliptical swelling of an indirect inguinal hernia descending into the scrotum on the right side. Also note the globular swelling of a direct inguinal hernia on the left side.
(b) To examine the inguinal canal in a male, invaginate the scrotum as shown (always wear gloves).

An **indirect inguinal hernia** passes through the internal inguinal ring, which lies 2 cm above the midpoint of the inguinal ligament, just above and lateral to the femoral pulse, and descends through the inguinal canal. In males a small indirect inguinal hernia may be palpated by gently invaginating the scrotum and feeling an impulse at the external ring when the patient coughs (see Fig 6.9(b)). When examining a male, remember to count the number of testes in the scrotum (normally two) as a maldescended testis may be confused with an inguinal hernia.

A **direct inguinal hernia** protrudes forwards through the inguinal (Hesselbach's) triangle. A direct inguinal hernia usually appears immediately with standing (and coughing or straining) and disappears on lying down.

Femoral hernias

A **femoral hernia** usually bulges *into the groin crease* at its *medial* end. Hence, these occur *lateral* to and *below* the pubic tubercle, 2 cm medial to the femoral pulse, and do not involve the inguinal canal. There may not be a cough impulse because of the presence of an omental plug or strangulation. Do not confuse an impulse conducted by the femoral vein (saphena varix) during coughing with a femoral hernia. A femoral hernia is usually small and firm and can be mistaken for a lymph node.

If a hernia strangulates, the overlying skin may become red and tense, and the lump is usually tender. The cough impulse is lost.

Remember that hernias are often bilateral, two different types may occur on the same side and there may be an associated **hydrocele** (increased fluid in the tunica vaginalis causing scrotal swelling). The upper end of a hydrocele is palpable in the inguinal canal, so you can get above a hydrocele in the inguinal canal but not a hernia.

Incisional hernias

Any abdominal scar may be the site of a hernia because of abdominal wall weakness. Assess this by asking the patient to cough while you look for abnormal bulges. Next have the patient lift his or her head and shoulders off the bed while your hand rests on the forehead and resists this movement. If a bulge is seen, your other hand should palpate for a fascial layer defect in the muscle.

Male genitalia

Inspect the scrotum for size and skin changes (e.g. ulceration). Palpate the scrotum for the **testes**. Feel each testis rather gently and note the size, regularity and firmness. The **spermatic cord** is palpable as it enters the scrotum: the **epididymis** on top of each testis is also usually palpable. There may be a mass in the scrotum separate from the testes. If it is not possible to find the upper limit of this mass it must have descended into the testis from above and is probably an inguinal hernia. A mass wholly within the testis should be tested for transillumination (see Fig 6.10) with a torch. A hydrocele is confined to the scrotum, will usually light up in an impressive manner, and the testis and epididymis are not palpable.

Bilateral **testicular atrophy** occurs in chronic liver disease (e.g. alcoholic liver disease, haemochromatosis).

Examine the **penis** if indicated. Put on gloves and inspect, looking for obvious rash, inflammation or a mass. Next palpate the glans penis through the foreskin, retract the foreskin (which is not possible in phimosis) and palpate the inguinal glands.

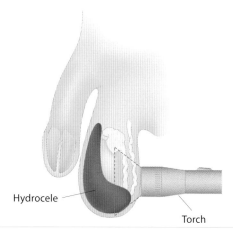

Hydrocele

Torch

Figure 6.10 Transillumination of the testes

Rectal examination

The abdominal examination is not complete without a rectal examination. Explain to the patient what is to happen, then lie the patient on his or her left side with the knees drawn up and the back facing you. This is called the left lateral position.

Don a pair of gloves and begin the inspection of the anus and perianal area by separating the buttocks. Note the presence of thrombosed external haemorrhoids (piles: small (< 1 cm), tense bluish swellings seen on one side of the anal margin) or skin tags (these look like tags elsewhere on the body and can be an incidental finding or occur with haemorrhoids or Crohn's disease).

The tip of the gloved right index finger is lubricated and placed over the anus. Ask the patient to breathe in and out quietly through the mouth, as a distraction and to aid relaxation. Slowly increasing pressure is applied with the pulp of the finger until the sphincter is felt to relax slightly. The finger is then advanced slowly into the rectum. At this stage sphincter tone should be assessed as increased, normal or reduced.

Palpation of the anterior wall of the rectum for the **prostate gland** in the male and for the cervix in the female is performed first. The normal prostate is a firm rubbery bilobed mass with a central furrow. The presence of a very hard nodule suggests carcinoma of the prostate is present. The prostate is boggy and tender in patients with prostatitis. The finger is then rotated clockwise so that the left lateral wall, posterior wall and right lateral wall of the rectum can be palpated in turn. Then the finger is advanced as high as possible into the rectum and slowly withdrawn along the rectal wall. After the finger has been withdrawn, the glove is inspected for bright blood or melaena, mucus or pus, and the colour of the faeces is noted.

Haemorrhoids are not palpable unless thrombosed. The occurrence of significant pain during the examination suggests an anal fissure, an ischiorectal abscess, a recently thrombosed external haemorrhoid, proctitis or anal ulceration.

Other signs in abdominal disease

General inspection

Look for jaundice (yellow sclerae), increased pigmentation (e.g. haemochromatosis), obesity or wasting (record the weight and height). Wasting may be due to malabsorption or malignancy (see box below).

Examining the patient with suspected malignancy

1 Palpate all draining lymph nodes.
2 Examine all remaining lymph node groups.
3 Examine the abdomen, particularly for hepatomegaly and ascites.
4 Feel the testes.
5 Perform a rectal examination and pelvic examination.
6 Examine the lungs.
7 Examine the breasts.
8 Examine the skin and nails (e.g. for melanoma).

Note any rashes. Fragile vesicles appear on exposed areas of the skin and heal with scarring in patients with porphyria cutanea tarda. The tense tethering of the skin in systemic sclerosis may be associated with gastro-oesophageal reflux and gastrointestinal motility disorders.

Look for the general signs of uraemia, including hyperventilation (metabolic acidosis), hiccupping, uraemic fetor (the breath smells rather like urine) and a sallow complexion.

Assess the state of hydration in all patients with suspected gastrointestinal or renal disease. Dehydration can be a cause of acute renal failure, while overhydration can result from intravenous infusions of fluid when attempts are made to correct acute renal failure.

The hands

Note any changes of **arthritis**. Arthropathy may be present in the hands in patients with the iron-storage disease, **haemochromatosis**.

Look for **purpura**, which is really any sort of bruising. The lesions can vary in size from pinheads called **petechiae** to large bruises called **ecchymoses**. If the petechiae are raised (**palpable purpura**), this suggests an underlying systemic vasculitis or bacteraemia.

At the **wrist** and **forearms**, inspect for **scars** and palpate for surgically created **arteriovenous fistulae** or **shunts** used for haemodialysis access. There is a longitudinal swelling and a palpable continuous thrill present over a fistula.

The nails

Leuconychia (white nails)
When chronic liver or other disease results in hypoalbuminaemia, the nail beds opacify, often leaving only a rim of pink nail bed at the top of the nail.

Clubbing
Up to one-third of patients with cirrhosis may have finger clubbing.

Koilonychia
These are dry, brittle, ridged, spoon-shaped nails due to severe iron-deficiency anaemia; they are rare these days.

The palms

Palmar erythema ('liver palms')
This is reddening of the palms of the hands affecting the thenar and hypothenar eminences. Often the soles of the feet are also affected. This can be a feature of chronic liver disease.

Anaemia
Inspect the palmar creases for pallor suggesting anaemia, which may result from gastrointestinal blood loss, malabsorption (folate, vitamin B_{12}), haemolysis (e.g. hypersplenism) or chronic systemic disease.

Dupuytren's contractures
This is a visible and palpable thickening and contraction of the palmar fascia causing permanent flexion, most often of the ring finger. It is often bilateral and occasionally may affect the feet. It is associated with alcoholism (not liver disease), but is also found in some manual workers; it may be familial.

Hepatic flap (asterixis)

Ask the patient to stretch out the arms in front, separate the fingers and extend the wrists for 15 seconds. Jerky, irregular flexion–extension movement at the wrist and metacarpophalangeal joints, often accompanied by lateral movements of the fingers, constitutes the flapping of hepatic encephalopathy in liver failure.

The arms

Inspect the upper limbs for **bruising**. Large bruises (ecchymoses) may be due to clotting abnormalities (e.g. in chronic liver disease).

Look for **muscle wasting**, which is often a late manifestation of malnutrition in alcoholic patients. Alcohol can also cause a proximal myopathy.

Scratch marks due to severe itch (pruritus) are often prominent in patients with obstructive or cholestatic jaundice.

Examine the **epitrochlear nodes**. Place the palm of the left hand under the patient's right elbow. Your thumb can then be placed over the node that is proximal and slightly anterior to the medial epicondyle. This is repeated with the right hand for the other side (see Fig 6.11).

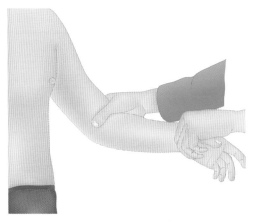

Figure 6.11 Feeling for the epitrochlear lymph node

Spider naevi consist of a central arteriole from which radiate numerous small vessels that look like spiders' legs. They range in size from just visible to 0.5 cm in diameter. Their usual distribution is in the area drained by the superior vena cava, so they are found on the arms, neck and chest wall. Pressure applied with a pointed object to the central arteriole causes blanching of the whole lesion. Rapid refilling occurs on release of the pressure.

The finding of more than two spider naevi anywhere on the body is likely to be abnormal except during pregnancy. Spider naevi are often caused by cirrhosis, most frequently due to alcohol.

Spider naevi can easily be distinguished from **Campbell de Morgan spots**, which are flat or slightly elevated red circular spots that occur on the abdomen or the front of the chest. They do not blanch on pressure and are very common and harmless.

Axillae

The axillary lymph nodes are palpated by raising the patient's arm and, using the left hand for the right side, push your fingers as high as possible into the axilla. The patient's arm is then brought down to rest on your forearm. The opposite is done for the other side (see Fig 6.12). There are five main groups of axillary nodes: (1) central; (2) lateral (above and lateral); (3) pectoral (medial); (4) infraclavicular; and (5) subscapular (most inferior). An effort should be made to feel for nodes in each of these areas of the axilla.

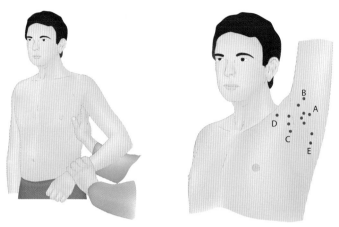

Figure 6.12 Feeling for the axillary lymph nodes: A = central, B = lateral, C = pectoral, D = infraclavicular, E = subscapular

Cervical and supraclavicular nodes

Sit the patient up and examine the cervical nodes from behind. There are eight groups. Attempt to identify each of the groups of nodes with your fingers (see Fig 6.13). First palpate the **submental** node, which lies directly under the chin, then the **submandibular** nodes, which are below the angle of the jaw. Next palpate the **jugular chain**, which lies anterior to the sternomastoid muscle, and then the **posterior triangle** nodes, which are posterior to the sternomastoid muscle. Palpate the **occipital** region for occipital nodes and then move to the **postauricular** node behind the ear and the **preauricular** node in front of the ear. Finally from the back, with the patient's shoulders slightly shrugged, feel in the supraclavicular fossa and at the base of the sternomastoid muscle for the **supraclavicular** nodes.

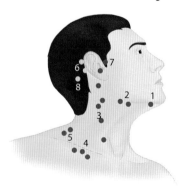

Figure 6.13 Cervical and supraclavicular nodes: 1 = submental, 2 = submandibular, 3 = jugular chain, 4 = supraclavicular, 5 = posterior triangle, 6 = postauricular, 7 = preauricular, 8 = occipital

The face

Eyes

Look first at the sclerae for signs of **jaundice** or **anaemia**. A red eye (**iritis**) may be seen in inflammatory bowel disease. **Conjunctival pallor** suggests anaemia. The most objective sign is to look for **conjunctival rim pallor**. In health, the anterior rim of the inferior conjunctiva is bright red; if it is pale, this has high diagnostic utility for anaemia compared with other physical signs, such as nail bed or palm crease pallor.

The salivary glands

The normal **parotid gland** is impalpable; enlargement leads to a swelling in the cheek behind the angle of the jaw and in the upper neck. Examine for signs of inflammation (warmth, tenderness, redness and swelling) and decide whether the facial swelling is lumpy or not (see Fig 6.14). A mixed parotid tumour (a pleomorphic adenoma) is the most common cause of a lump. Alcoholic liver disease can cause bilateral swelling. Mumps also causes acute parotid enlargement, which is usually bilateral. Parotid carcinoma may cause a facial nerve palsy (p. 121). Feel in the mouth (wear a glove!) for a parotid calculus, which may be present at the parotid duct orifice (opposite the upper second molar).

Submandibular gland enlargement is most often due to a calculus. This may be palpable bimanually. Place your index finger on the floor of the patient's mouth beside the tongue, feeling between it and fingers placed behind the body of the mandible. It may also be enlarged in chronic liver disease.

The mouth

The teeth and breath

Look first briefly at the state of the teeth and note whether they are real or false. False teeth will have to be removed for complete examination of the mouth. Loose-fitting false teeth may be responsible for ulcers, and decayed teeth may be responsible for bad breath (fetor). **Fetor hepaticus** is a sweet smell of the breath and is an indication of hepatocellular failure.

The tongue

Thickened epithelium with bacterial debris and food particles commonly cause a **coating** over the tongue, especially in smokers. It is rarely a sign of disease.

Leucoplakia is white-coloured thickening of the mucosa of the tongue and mouth; the condition is premalignant. Most of the causes of leucoplakia begin with 'S'—sore teeth (poor dental hygiene), smoking, spirits, sepsis or syphilis—but often no cause is apparent.

The term **glossitis** is generally used to describe a smooth appearance of the tongue, which may also be erythematous. The appearance is due to atrophy of the papillae, and in later stages there may be shallow ulceration. These changes occur in the tongue often as a result of nutritional deficiencies (e.g. vitamin B_{12}, folate or iron).

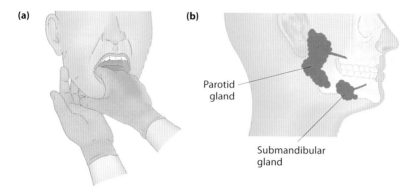

(a) **(b)**

Parotid
gland

Submandibular
gland

Figure 6.14 (a) Examination of the parotid gland   **(b)** The salivary glands

Oral cavity

Aphthous ulceration is common. It begins as a small painful vesicle on the tongue or mucosal surface of the mouth, which may break down to form a painful shallow ulcer with surrounding erythema. These ulcers heal without scarring. They usually do not indicate any serious underlying systemic disease, but may occur in Crohn's disease or coeliac disease.

Fungal infection with *Candida albicans* (thrush) causes creamy white, curd-like patches in the mouth or on the tongue, which are removed only with difficulty and leave a bleeding surface. These can be associated with immune deficiency (e.g. human immunodeficiency virus (HIV) infection).

Look for hypertrophy of the gums, which may occur with infiltration by leukaemic cells, especially in cases of acute monocytic leukaemia. Look next for gum bleeding, ulceration, infection or haemorrhage of the buccal and pharyngeal mucosa. Also look for telangiectasia (which may be a sign of hereditary haemorrhagic telangiectasia that causes occult bleeding in the bowel).

The chest

In males, **gynaecomastia** or enlargement of the breasts may be a sign of chronic liver disease. Tender gynaecomastia is common when patients take the drug spironolactone.

The back

Strike the vertebral column gently with the base of the fist to elicit bony tenderness. This may be due to malignant deposits. Look for sacral oedema in a patient confined to bed (e.g. from nephrotic syndrome or congestive cardiac failure).

The legs

Note oedema, purpura, pigmentation or scratch marks. **Pruritus** (itch) may be associated with renal failure and obstructive jaundice because toxins are deposited in the skin.

Leg ulcers may occur above the medial or lateral malleolus in association with haemolytic anaemia (including sickle cell anaemia and hereditary spherocytosis). Tender, raised ulcerated areas on the legs (**pyoderma gangrenosum**) are an important but uncommon sign of inflammatory bowel disease.

Look for the neurological signs of alcoholism (e.g. a coarse tremor) or evidence of thiamine deficiency (peripheral neuropathy or memory loss), which may also be present (p. 142).

The fundi

Look for engorged retinal vessels and papilloedema. This can occur in diseases such as macroglobulinaemia, which increase blood viscosity. Haemorrhages may occur with severe thrombocytopenia, especially when it is associated with anaemia.

Urinalysis

The urine can be tested with a dip stick for certain abnormalities. Colour changes on the stick will indicate pH, protein (proteinuria), sugar (diabetes mellitus), nitrites (possible infection) and red blood cells (haematuria).

The abdomen OSCE: hints panel

1 **This man has noticed that his sclerae have turned yellow. Take a history from him.**
   (a) This is likely to be jaundice (which should be obvious on inspection). Ask him the following:
      (i) Have you noticed a change in the colour of your skin and of the whites of your eyes?
      (ii) How long has it been present? Is it getting better or worse? Has it happened before?
      (iii) Are you itchy?
      (iv) Has the colour of your urine or stools changed (dark urine and pale stools in obstructive jaundice)?
      (v) Have you lost weight (e.g. malignancy involving the liver or pancreas)?
      (vi) Do you have any abdominal pain? Ask about the symptoms of biliary colic.
      (vii) Does your abdomen swell up (ascites)? Do you develop leg swelling (oedema)?
      (viii) Have you ever vomited blood or passed black stools (haematemesis and melaena—may be from bleeding oesophageal varices)?
      (ix) Have you ever had hepatitis?
      (x) Have you had fatigue, nausea, anorexia, myalgias, bruising?
      (xi) Do you now or have you in the past drunk large amounts of alcohol?
      (xii) Have you had a liver biopsy? Do you know what is wrong with your liver?
      (xiii) Do you suffer any memory loss or confusion (hepatic encephalopathy)?

(b) Does the patient have any history of blood transfusions, drug use, tattoos or body piercing (e.g. hepatitis C or B)?

(c) Take the sexual history.

(d) Take the medication history (drug-induced hepatitis).

(e) Check whether there is a family history of liver problems.

(f) Synthesise and present your findings.

2 **This woman has been diagnosed as having liver failure. Please examine her abdomen.**

(a) Ask the patient's permission to examine her abdomen and ask her to lie flat with her abdomen exposed from the lower ribs to the symphysis pubis.

(b) While the patient is undressing, stand back to look for obvious signs of chronic liver disease.

(c) Ask whether any part of her abdomen is tender and to let you know if any part of the examination is uncomfortable.

(d) Examine the abdomen systematically (inspect, palpate, percuss, auscultate). Assess particularly for ascites and hepatosplenomegaly.

(e) Ask whether you may examine other regions. Note any jaundice or scleral pallor (anaemia).

(f) Look for spider naevi and gynaecomastia on the chest wall (signs of chronic liver disease).

(g) Look for finger clubbing, leuconychia and palmar erythema (signs of chronic liver disease).

(h) Test for a liver flap and fetor hepaticus, and assess orientation and mental state (liver failure).

(i) Synthesise and present your findings.

3 **Please examine this man's abdomen. He has a family history of renal impairment and hypertension.**

(a) Ask the patient's permission to examine his abdomen and ask him to lie flat with his abdomen exposed from the lower ribs to the symphysis pubis.

(b) Look for abdominal distension.

(c) Ask about areas of tenderness.

(d) Examine the abdomen, paying particular attention to the palpation of the kidneys since the likely diagnosis is polycystic kidneys.

(e) Attempt to outline the size of the kidneys and detect the characteristic cystic shape.

(f) Ballotte the kidneys and demonstrate that you can get above them (i.e. that there is renal enlargement, not hepatosplenomegaly).

(g) Take the blood pressure.

(h) Synthesise and present your findings.

4 **This woman has a lymphoma. Please examine her abdomen.**

(a) Ask the patient's permission to examine her abdomen and ask her to lie flat with her abdomen exposed from the lower ribs to the symphysis pubis.

(b) While the patient is undressing, look for wasting, abdominal distension and surgical scars.

6

(c) Ask about tenderness or discomfort.

(d) Examine the abdomen. Pay particular attention to the size of the liver and spleen, and palpate for enlarged abdominal lymph nodes.

(e) Examine all the other lymph node groups, starting with the inguinal nodes.

(f) Ask whether you have time to examine the chest.

(g) Synthesise and present your findings.

5 This man has a hernia in the groin. Please examine him.

(a) Explain to the patient what you want to do and ask his permission.

(b) Get him to stand in front of you and remove his underpants.

(c) Inspect the groins for lumps.

(d) Try to decide whether the lump is an inguinal or a femoral hernia by palpation of its position.

(e) Gently push it back into the abdomen. Is it reducible?

(f) Ask the patient to cough and feel for a cough impulse.

(g) Wearing gloves, invaginate the scrotum gently and feel for the external ring and an impulse as the patient coughs.

(h) Note the number of testes in the scrotum.

(i) Synthesise and present your findings.

6 This man has found a lump in his neck. Please examine his lymph nodes.

(a) Ask the patient to remove his shirt and sit up over the edge of the bed.

(b) Stand back to look for wasting or obvious scars or abdominal distension.

(c) Examine the epitrochlear, axillary and cervical (including supraclavicular) nodes with him in this position. Keep in mind the characteristics of different lymph node abnormalities.

(d) Next lay the patient flat and expose the abdomen.

(e) Feel for para-aortic and inguinal nodes, for splenomegaly and for hepatomegaly.

(f) If a group of nodes is abnormal, consider their area of drainage and ask to examine that region. If many groups are enlarged, consider a lymphoma as the cause.

(g) Synthesise and present your findings.

The abdominal history and examination

hints for success

1 Eliciting individual gastrointestinal symptoms and the pattern of presentation will often lead to the correct diagnosis.

2 The symptoms and signs of renal disease may be non-specific.

3 Abnormal bruising or bleeding tendencies should be asked about as a routine.

4 When examining the abdomen, it is important to position the patient flat. While palpating, consider the underlying organs that are present when abnormalities are detected.

5 If an abdominal mass is found, characterise it, then pay special attention to the liver, rectal examination and supraclavicular nodes.

continued

6   A left upper quadrant mass may be a spleen or kidney. Remember that one cannot get above the spleen and that the spleen is not ballottable.

7   An inguinal hernia bulges above the crease of the groin, whereas a femoral hernia bulges into the medial end of the groin crease.

8   Lymphadenopathy is a major sign of haematological disease or malignancy and all lymph node groups must be examined carefully.

9   A gastrointestinal system examination is incomplete without a rectal examination.

10 Examination of the urine is an important extension of the physical examination.

chapter 7

The nervous system

Brain: That collection of vessels and organs in the head, from which sense and motion arise.

S Johnson, *A Dictionary Of The English Language* (1755)

Neurological history taking and examination require an approach that is very systematic and thorough. Only by this means can the symptoms and signs be assembled in a way that will enable a sensible neurological diagnosis.

The neurological system assessment sequence

1 Presenting symptoms, e.g. headache, syncope, dizziness, sensory changes, motor weakness, balance problems
2 Detailed questions about the presenting symptoms and especially their time course (SOCRATES, p. 4)
3 Questions about previous neurological problems and risk factors (e.g. family history, hypertension, medications), results of precious investigations and handedness
4 General examination for orientation and level of consciousness, and neck stiffness
5 A general inspection for wasting, tremor or abnormal movements
6 Examination of the cranial nerves (including fundi).
7 Examination of the motor system and reflexes (including gait).
8 Sensory system examination, directed by the history and other examination findings
9 Provisional and differential diagnosis

The neurological history

Presenting symptoms (see Table 7.1)

The **temporal course of a neurological illness** usually gives important information about the underlying aetiology. An acute onset of symptoms suggests a vascular problem, a subacute onset suggests an inflammatory disorder, and a more chronic symptom course suggests that the underlying disorder may be related to either a tumour or a degenerative process. Metabolic or toxic disorders may present with any of these patterns. Episodic or recurrent symptoms may be vascular (e.g. transient ischaemic attacks or migraines) or due to vestibular disease.

A judgement must also be made as to whether the disease process is **localised** or **diffuse**, and what levels of the nervous system are involved.

Table 7.1 Neurological history
Presenting symptoms
Headache
Facial pain
Back or neck pain
Fits, faints or funny turns
Vertigo or dizziness
Disturbances of vision, hearing or smell
Disturbances of gait
Loss of or disturbed sensation, or weakness in a limb(s)
Disturbances of sphincter control (bladder, bowels)
Involuntary movements or tremor
Speech and swallowing disturbance
Altered cognition (see Table 7.2)
Risk factors for cerebrovascular disease
Hypertension
Smoking
Diabetes mellitus
Hyperlipidaemia
Atrial fibrillation, bacterial endocarditis, valvular heart disease
Bleeding disorders, anticoagulant drugs, thrombophilic disorders
Family history of stroke

Headache and facial pain

Headache is a common and difficult symptom but the diagnosis may be clear once the pattern has been determined.

Tension-type headache may be episodic or chronic, commonly bilateral, and occurs over the frontal, occipital or temporal areas. It may be described as a sensation of tightness. These headaches last for hours, recur often and lack the specific features of other headaches. This is the most common type.

Classical migraine is usually a unilateral headache preceded by an aura (e.g. flashing lights) and is commonly associated with photophobia (light intolerance). It is often of incapacitating severity and associated with nausea and vomiting. **Common migraine** is a similar headache without the other neurological symptoms and is, of course, much more common.

Cluster headache is a severe, steady boring pain behind or over one eye lasting 15 minutes to 2 hours, associated with lacrimation, rhinorrhoea and flushing of the forehead. It tends to occur at the same time each day, often at night.

Cervical spondylosis can cause headache over the occiput that is associated with neck pain.

Raised intracranial pressure results in generalised headache that is worse in the morning and may be associated with drowsiness or vomiting and progressive neurological deficits.

Meningitis causes generalised headache associated with photophobia, fever and a stiff neck.

Temporal arteritis causes persistent headache, usually over the temporal area associated with tenderness over the temporal artery. There may be jaw claudication (pain on eating or talking) as well as acute visual loss.

Acute sinusitis headache is associated with pain or fullness behind the eyes or over the cheeks or forehead.

Subarachnoid haemorrhage characteristically causes dramatic and usually instantaneous onset of severe headache.

Faints and fits

Transient loss of consciousness may have a neurological cause but cardiac arrhythmias and metabolic diseases are other possible explanations. The following should be considered.

Syncope due to a simple faint is the most common cause of loss of consciousness. The episode is usually very brief and is often preceded by pallor, sweating, nausea and dizziness. If the degree of cerebral hypoperfusion is severe, there may be a few clonic jerks or a brief tonic spasm ('convulsive syncope'). There tends to be minimal confusion following the episode.

Epilepsy is an abrupt loss of consciousness, which may be preceded by an aura—an abnormal sensation (e.g. a hallucination involving one of the senses, or altered cognition such as a sense of deja vu). Bystanders may have observed tonic (sustained contraction of the muscles for 20–30 seconds) and clonic (violent rhythmical) movements. However, cerebral hypoxia of any cause (e.g. from severe bradycardia) can cause these movements. The patient who has had a major seizure may sleep for a period after the episode and may wake to find that he or she has bitten the tongue and been incontinent.

Transient ischaemic attacks affect the brain stem. These may rarely cause loss of consciousness without warning.

Hypoglycaemia usually occurs in diabetic patients on insulin or taking oral hypoglycaemic drugs. These patients may feel anxious, sweaty and notice a fast heart rate before unconsciousness occurs—these are autonomic nervous system responses to hypoglycaemia.

Hysteria may cause bizarre attacks of apparent loss of consciousness.

Vertigo and dizziness

In true **vertigo**, there is actually a sense of motion. The world seems to turn around. This can be caused by vestibular disease (acute labyrinthitis, benign positional vertigo or Ménière's disease) or cerebellar disease (such as that caused by alcohol, anticonvulsants, multiple sclerosis, vascular lesions or tumour). **Dizziness** can be a feeling of impending unconsciousness or merely of momentary unsteadiness.

Disturbances of vision, hearing or smell

These symptoms may reflect a cranial nerve lesion. Ask about double vision (diplopia), blurred vision, loss of vision (amblyopia) and light intolerance (photophobia). Ask also about loss of hearing in one or both ears, and about ringing in the ears (tinnitus).

Disturbances of gait

Many neurological conditions can make walking difficult. **Cerebellar disease** makes walking unsteady and uncertain. **Hemiplegia** after a stroke makes walking difficult because of an increase in tone and loss of power in the affected leg. A **peripheral neuropathy** or spinal cord disease may alter position sense in the legs. Parkinson's disease causes a characteristic shuffling gait. Hysteria can also present with a bizarrely abnormal gait. Walking may also be abnormal when orthopaedic disease affects the lower limbs or spine.

Disturbed sensation or weakness in the limbs

Pins and needles in the hands or feet more often indicates nerve entrapment or a peripheral neuropathy but can result from sensory pathway involvement at any level.

Limb weakness may be due to cerebral, spinal cord (including anterior horn cell), nerve root, peripheral nerve, neuromuscular junction or muscle disease. Distinguishing between an upper and lower motor neuron lesion is important (see box on pp. 122–3).

Autonomic symptoms

Ask about bladder or bowel incontinence, impotence (in men) or postural dizziness, all of which may be symptoms of autonomic neuropathy.

Tremor and involuntary movements

Tremors are fine involuntary repetitive movements. **Action tremors** are worse when a voluntary movement is attempted. These include an enhanced physiological tremor, as may occur in essential tremors, anxiety and thyrotoxicosis. **Intention** (or **target seeking) tremor** becomes worse as the limb gets closer to an object reached for and is due to cerebellar disease. Parkinson's disease may present with a **resting tremor** (characteristically a 'pill rolling' tremor) while in **chorea** there are irregular jerky movements.

Past health

Enquire about a past history of meningitis or encephalitis, head or spinal injuries and epilepsy, or risk factors for human immunodeficiency virus

(HIV) infection or syphilis, which may have nervous system involvement. Anticonvulsant drugs, the contraceptive pill, antihypertensive agents, chemotherapeutic agents, anti-Parkinsonian drugs, steroids, anticoagulants and anti-platelet agents may be used for neurological conditions or may have neurological effects and need to be documented. Ask about risk factors that may predispose to the development of cerebrovascular disease (see Table 7.1).

Social history

As smoking predisposes to cerebrovascular disease, the smoking history is relevant. It is also useful to ask about occupation and exposure to toxins (e.g. heavy metals, pesticides). Alcohol intake can also result in a number of neurological diseases, such as cerebellar degeneration, short-term memory impairment and peripheral neuropathy.

Family history

Any history of neurological or mental disease should be documented.

The mental state examination

Any patient who has a history of confusion, or is suspected of having dementia or a major psychiatric illness, should undergo a mental state examination. A rapid way of testing for orientation, memory and attention is to have the patient complete a mini-mental state examination (see Table 7.2). Even gross disturbances of these functions may not be obvious unless they are formally tested.

Table 7.2 **The mini-mental state examination**		
	Score	**Max**
Orientation		
'What is the (year) (season) (date) (month)?' Ask for the date, then specifically enquire about the parts omitted (e.g. seasons). Score 1 point for each correct answer.	☐	5
'Where are we (country) (state) (town) (hospital) (ward)?' Ask in turn for each place. Score 1 point for each correct answer.	☐	5
Registration		
'May I test your memory?' Repeat three objects (e.g. pen, watch, book). Score 1 point for each correct answer. Then repeat until the patient learns all three. Count trials and record (up to six).	☐	3

continued

Table 7.2 **The mini-mental state examination** *continued*

Attention and calculation

'Count backwards from 100 by sevens' (Serial 7s). Score 1 point for each answer, up to five (93, 86, 79, 72, 65). Or Spell 'world' backwards. Score 1 point for each letter in correct order.	☐	5

Recall

Ask the patient to recall the three objects in 'Registration' (above). Score 1 point for each correct answer.	☐	3

Language

Ask the patient to name two objects shown (e.g. pen and watch). Score 0–2 points.	☐	2
'Repeat the following: 'No ifs, ands or buts'. Score 1 point.	☐	1
Ask the patient to follow a three-stage command: e.g. 'Take this paper in your right hand, fold it in half and put it on the table.' Score 1 point for each step.	☐	3
Read and obey the following: CLOSE YOUR EYES. Score 1 point.	☐	1
WRITE A SENTENCE. Do not dictate—it must be sensible, but punctuation and grammar are not essential. Score 1 point.	☐	1
COPY THIS DESIGN. All ten angles must be present, and the two must intersect. Score 1 point.	☐	1
Total	☐	30

Assess the patient's level of consciousness along a continuum:

Alert   Drowsy   Stuporous   Coma

A score of 21–29 indicates mild cognitive impairment.
A score below 20 indicates more severe cognitive impairment, and is highly likely to be due to dementia, especially if obtained on repeated examinations.

Neurological examination technique

The neurological examination is complicated but rewarding. Adequate interpretation of neurological signs requires an understanding of basic neuroanatomy. The following components must be systematically assessed:

1. **General.** This includes examination for the level of consciousness, the presence of neck stiffness, and the assessment of speech and the higher centres.
2. **The cranial nerves.** Examine the cranial nerves II (including the fundi) to XII. The first (olfactory) nerve is often omitted but anosmia (absence of ability to smell) may be the only sign of a frontal meningioma.
3. **The upper limbs.** Assessment involves:
   * **motor system:** inspection, tone, power, reflexes and coordination
   * **sensory system:** pain (pinprick) sensation, light touch, proprioception (position sense) and vibration sense.
4. **The lower limbs.** Assess as for the upper limbs (motor and sensory systems) but include an assessment of walking (gait).
5. **The skull and spine.** Assess for local disease, if relevant.
6. **The carotid arteries.** Auscultate both sides for bruits. There may be no bruit with severe carotid stenosis (> 90% blockage). It may not be possible to diagnose a separate carotid bruit in patients with aortic stenosis.

Neck stiffness and Kernig's sign

This examination is absolutely essential for any febrile or acutely ill patient, or for anyone with altered mental status. Slip one hand under the patient's head and attempt to gently flex the head so that the patient's chin touches the chest (see Fig 7.1). Resistance due to painful spasm of the extensor muscles of the neck will occur if the meninges are inflamed. Next, flex the patient's hip and then attempt to straighten the patient's knee. Painful spasm of the hamstrings will occur if there is inflammation around the lumbar spinal roots—**Kernig's sign** (see Fig 7.2).

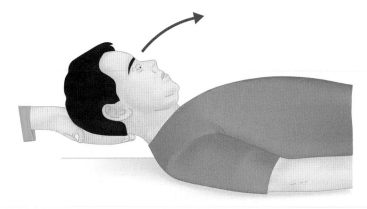

Figure 7.1 Testing for neck stiffness

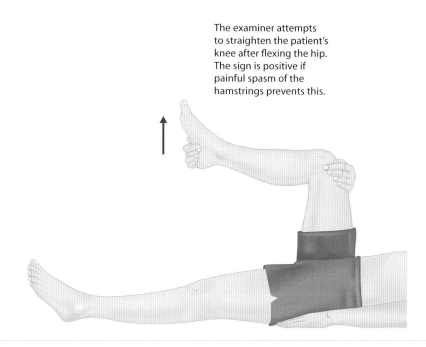

The examiner attempts to straighten the patient's knee after flexing the hip. The sign is positive if painful spasm of the hamstrings prevents this.

Figure 7.2 Kernig's sign

Handedness, orientation, speech and higher centres

Ask the patient whether he or she is right- or left-handed (to help determine the likely dominant hemisphere, which is in the left brain in most right-handed people).

As a screening assessment, ask for the patient's name, present location and the date. This tests **orientation** in person, place and time. These tests are part of the mini-mental state examination (see Table 7.2).

Next ask the patient to name an object pointed at, then ask the patient to point to a named object in the room. This screens for dysphasia (**receptive dysphasia**—inability to understand speech; **expressive dysphasia**—inability to answer appropriately; **nominal dysphasia**—inability to name objects; or **conductive dysphasia**—inability to repeat speech) (see box below).

Dysarthria is a problem with the mechanical production of speech. Ask the patient to say 'West Register Street' or 'British Constitution'. This is a test for cerebellar dysfunction and its effect on speech. Cerebellar disease (and acute alcoholic intoxication) causes slurring and staccato speech. Next ask the patient to count to 30 to determine whether the muscles fatigue, which can also cause dysarthria (e.g. myasthenia gravis).

Dysphonia refers to impaired sound production from the larynx. Ask the patient to say 'Aaah' and to cough.

Examination of a patient with dysphasia

Wernicke's area in the superior posterior **temporal lobe** of the dominant cerebral hemisphere comprehends speech. A lesion here causes **receptive (sensory) dysphasia**.

Broca's area in the inferior **frontal lobe** of the dominant cerebral hemisphere controls language expression. A lesion here causes **expressive (motor) dysphasia.**

The **arcuate fasciculus** connects Wernicke's and Broca's areas. A lesion here causes **conduction dysphasia**.

Fluent speech (receptive or conduction dysphasia)

1 *Naming objects.* Patients with conduction and receptive dysphasia will name objects poorly. In nominal dysphasia, this is the only abnormality (dominant posterior temporoparietal lesion).
2 *Repetition.* Patients with conductive and receptive dysphasia have difficult repeating words or phrases.
3 *Comprehension.* Receptive dysphasic patients cannot follow commands (verbal or written). In conduction dysphasia commands can be followed.

Non-fluent speech (expressive dysphasia)

1 *Naming objects.* This is absent or poor but may be better than spontaneous speech.
2 *Repetition.* This may be possible with great effort. Phrase repetition (e.g. 'No ifs, ands or buts') is poor.
3 *Comprehension.* This is relatively normal, and written and verbal commands can be followed.
4 *Reading.* Patients may have dyslexia.
5 *Writing.* Dysgraphia may be present.
6 *Look for hemiparesis* (upper motor neuron weakness on one side). The arm is more affected than the leg (p. 125).

Cranial nerves

The patient should be sat over the edge of the bed if possible. Begin with a general inspection of the head and neck. Look for **craniotomy** scars, which suggest previous surgery that has required opening of the skull. Then examine the cranial nerves in roughly the order of their number (see Fig 7.3). The use of a systematic approach is the only way to be sure nothing important is left out.

The first (olfactory) nerve

Testing is not performed routinely but is required if there is suspected loss of smell (anosmia). Each nostril is tested separately using non-pungent substances in a series of sample bottles. The patient sniffs these delicately and should be able to identify common smells, such as coffee and vanilla.

The second (optic) nerve (see also Ch 8)

Always test **visual acuity** with the patient wearing his or her reading spectacles, if required. Each eye is tested separately, while the other is

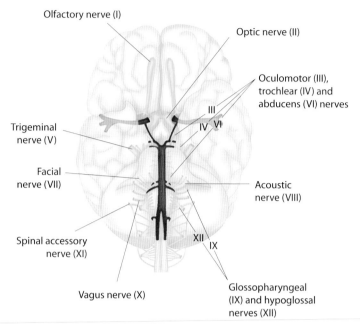

Olfactory nerve (I)

Optic nerve (II)

Oculomotor (III), trochlear (IV) and abducens (VI) nerves

III

IV VI

Trigeminal nerve (V)

Facial nerve (VII)

Acoustic nerve (VIII)

Spinal accessory nerve (XI)

XII

IX

Vagus nerve (X)

Glossopharyngeal (IX) and hypoglossal nerves (XII)

Figure 7.3 The location of the cranial nerves

covered with a small card. The patient is asked to read letters on a chart. The standard chart is read reflected in a mirror from 3 m away (effectively 6 m). The ability to read the letters normally visible at this distance is called 6/6 vision. The ability only to read larger letters normally visible at 60 m is called 6/60 vision. A hand-held chart can be carried and used as an alternative. Patients with poor visual acuity may only be able to distinguish hand movements or light and dark.

Examine the **visual fields**. One method involves confrontation with a red-topped hatpin. In this examination the patient's field of vision is compared with yours (see Fig 7.4(a)). Your head should be level with the patient's head. You can use your finger to test the visual fields (as shown in Fig 7.4(a)). Move your left or right finger in each visual field and ask the patient which finger has moved. A more sensitive method is to test each eye separately with the other eye covered. Slowly bring the pin into each quadrant diagonally. When the pin is brought into your visual field and the patient's, it should become visible to both of you at the same point. You must watch for the pin and also watch the patient's eye to ensure that it remains looking straight ahead. Patients are often tempted to look towards the pin. A number of visual field defects can be detected, as shown in Figure 7.4(b).

If visual acuity is poor, the fields are mapped using the fingers instead of a pin. Ask the patient to say when your first and second fingers become visible as they are brought into the quadrants of the visual fields.

Look into the **fundi** (p. 147).

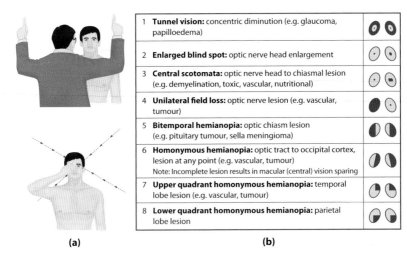

1	**Tunnel vision:** concentric diminution (e.g. glaucoma, papilloedema)	
2	**Enlarged blind spot:** optic nerve head enlargement	
3	**Central scotomata:** optic nerve head to chiasmal lesion (e.g. demyelination, toxic, vascular, nutritional)	
4	**Unilateral field loss:** optic nerve lesion (e.g. vascular, tumour)	
5	**Bitemporal hemianopia:** optic chiasm lesion (e.g. pituitary tumour, sella meningioma)	
6	**Homonymous hemianopia:** optic tract to occipital cortex, lesion at any point (e.g. vascular, tumour) Note: Incomplete lesion results in macular (central) vision sparing	
7	**Upper quadrant homonymous hemianopia:** temporal lobe lesion (e.g. vascular, tumour)	
8	**Lower quadrant homonymous hemianopia:** parietal lobe lesion	

(a)   (b)

Figure 7.4 (a) Testing the visual fields by confrontation. Compare your visual fields with those of the patient (both eyes, then cover one eye) and watch the patient to ensure the patient's eye is staring directly ahead.
(b) Visual field defects associated with lesions of the visual system

The third (oculomotor), fourth (trochlear) and sixth (abducens) nerves

These nerves control eye movements, the upper eyelid and pupil size, and are usually tested together. Look at the pupils, noting the shape, relative sizes and any associated ptosis (complete or partial involuntary eyelid closure).

If one pupil, or both pupils, is small this is called **miosis**. Causes include eye drops for glaucoma, narcotics, Horner's syndrome (interruption of the sympathetic innervation of the eye, which also causes ptosis of the eyelid), a pontine brain haemorrhage and, rarely, syphilis—the Argyll Robertson pupil.

Enlargement of the pupils is called **mydriasis**. Causes include a third nerve palsy (unilateral) and instillation of mydriatic eye drops. Other causes include Adie's pupil (a ciliary ganglion lesion), trauma and iritis with synechiae. Unequal pupils may be physiological and this condition is called **essential anisocoria**.

Use a pocket torch and shine the light from the side to gauge the **reaction** of the pupils to light. Assess quickly both the normal **direct** (constriction of the illuminated pupil) and normal **consensual** (constriction of the other pupil) responses. Remember that *both* pupils should normally contract briskly and equally when a light is shone into one.

Test **accommodation** (the constriction of the pupils that occurs when the eyes focus on a near object) by asking the patient to look into the distance and then at an object (e.g. a hatpin or a pen) placed about 20 cm from the nose.

Assess **eye movements** with both eyes first, getting the patient to follow the pin or finger laterally right and left, then up and down (in an H pattern).

Look for failure of movement (remember that the lateral rectus muscle, supplied by the sixth nerve, only moves the eye horizontally outwards; see Fig 8.2). Ask about **diplopia** (double vision) and in which direction of gaze the diplopia is most pronounced. Diplopia may be due to weakness of one or more of the ocular muscles. The separation of the images is greatest in the direction in which the affected muscle has its dominant effect.

Look for **nystagmus**. This is really an involuntary rhythmic oscillation of the ocular muscles back and forth. It may be *pendular* where the oscillations of the eye occur centrally and are equal in each direction. This usually indicates a problem with fixation. **Phasic** (jerky) **nystagmus** involves a slow drifting movement and a rapid correcting movement. The direction of the nystagmus is defined as the direction of the fast phase. Phasic nystagmus is a sign of cerebellar, brain stem or vestibular disease. Fine phasic nystagmus is normal at the extremes of gaze, so testing should involve asking the patient to follow your finger so that each eye is abducted about 30° in turn.

Remember the characteristic signs of palsies of the third, fourth and fifth nerves:

- *third nerve:* ipsilateral (same side as the lesion) mydriasis that is unreactive to light or accommodation, complete ptosis and divergent strabismus (the eye is deviated down and out)
- *fourth nerve:* inability to turn the eye down and in; the patient's head may be tilted away from the abnormal side
- *sixth nerve:* failure of lateral movement, with diplopia most pronounced on looking laterally on the affected side.

The fifth (trigeminal) nerve

Test the **corneal reflexes** gently using a wisp of cottonwool to touch the cornea and ask the patient whether the touch can be felt. Normally *both* the eyelids should shut briskly. The sensory component of this reflex is the fifth nerve and the motor component is the seventh nerve.

Test **facial sensation** in the three divisions: ophthalmic, maxillary and mandibular (see Fig 7.5). Test **pain** (pinprick) **sensation** with a new disposable neurology pin or blunt cannulae in each area. Start on one side of the forehead and move to the other side, pressing the pin into the skin and asking the patient to tell you what he or she feels (sharp is normal!). Map any area of sensory loss. If areas of reduced sensation (dull) are found, map them by moving the pin until normal sensation is again present (sharp). Test **light touch** by touching but not stroking the skin with a piece of cottonwool.

Note the presence of **sensory dissociation** (usually loss of pain and temperature sensation and preservation of light touch). This is rare but occurs typically in syringobulbia, where enlargement of the central canal of the brain stem and upper spinal cord interrupts crossing pain and temperature fibres first.

Examine the **motor** division of the fifth nerve by asking the patient to **clench** the teeth while you feel the masseter muscles. Then get the patient to **open** his or her mouth while you attempt to **force it closed**; this is not

7

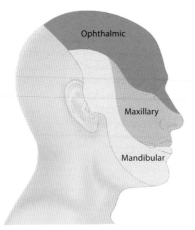

Figure 7.5 The divisions of the trigeminal nerve

possible if the pterygoid muscles are working. A unilateral lesion causes the jaw to deviate towards the weak (affected) side because the normal muscle's action is unopposed.

Test the **jaw jerk** by tapping the reflex hammer on your own thumb placed on the chin of the patient, whose mouth is partly open. This is present in normal people but is exaggerated, with brisk bilateral contraction of the masseter muscles, in cases of pseudobulbar palsy (bilateral upper motor neuron lesions also affecting the ninth, tenth and twelfth nerves) (see p. 122).

The seventh (facial) nerve

Test the muscles of **facial expression**. Ask the patient to look up and *wrinkle the forehead*. Look for loss of wrinkling and feel the muscle strength by pushing down on each side. This is preserved in an upper motor neuron lesion because of bilateral cortical representation of these muscles.

Next ask the patient to *shut his or her eyes tightly* and compare the two sides. Both upper and lower unilateral facial weakness can lead to incomplete closure of the eye on the same side, but a lower motor neuron lesion has a more pronounced effect. Tell the patient to *grin* and *compare the nasolabial grooves*. The side on which the groove is less pronounced is the abnormal one.

The eighth (acoustic) nerve

Quantitative hearing assessment is not possible without special equipment, but useful qualitative information can be obtained at the bedside. Whisper a number 60 cm away from each of the patient's ears while the other ear is distracted by movement of your finger near the auditory canal. It takes practice to know at what level of loudness a whisper is normally audible.

If there is deafness, perform **Rinné's** and **Weber's** tests and examine the external auditory canals and the eardrums (see Ch 8).

The ninth (glossopharyngeal) and tenth (vagus) nerves

Look at the palate and note any **uvular displacement**. Ask the patient to say 'ah' and look for symmetrical movement of the soft palate. With a unilateral lesion of the tenth nerve the uvula is drawn towards the unaffected (normal) side.

It may be unwise to test even gently for a **gag reflex** (the **ninth** nerve is the sensory component and the **tenth** nerve the motor component), whereby a spatula is touched onto each side of the soft palate in turn. The normal response is gagging with contraction of the palate on both sides, or even vomiting. To test the sensory (afferent) limb of the reflex, it is preferable to **touch the pharynx on each side**, and ask whether the touch can be felt and seems the same on each side. The motor (efferent) limb of this reflex would have been tested when the patient said 'ah'.

Ask the patient to speak to assess **hoarseness**, and to cough and to swallow. A 'bovine' or hollow cough suggests bilateral recurrent laryngeal nerve lesions.

The eleventh (accessory) nerve

Ask the patient to shrug his or her shoulders and feel the **trapezius** as you push the shoulders down. Then ask the patient to turn his or her head against resistance and feel the bulk of the **sternomastoid**. The normal muscle turns the head to the opposite side. Nerve palsy (a lower motor neuron lesion) causes weak contraction of the sternomastoid muscle ipsilateral to the lesion (i.e. weakness of head turning to the opposite side). An upper motor neuron lesion may cause weakness of contralateral head version because of ipsilateral sternomastoid weakness.

The twelfth (hypoglossal) nerve

While examining the mouth inspect the **tongue** for **wasting** and **fasciculation** (random flickering movements of small muscle groups), which is characteristic of a lower motor neuron lesion. Next ask the patient to **protrude the tongue**. A unilateral lesion causes the tongue to deviate towards the weaker (affected) side.

Upper versus lower motor neuron lesions

Remember the difference between upper and lower motor neuron lesions (see Figs 7.6 and 7.7). A lesion that interrupts the neural pathway above the anterior horn cell in the spinal cord is called an **upper motor neuron lesion**. Examples include lesions of the cortex, internal capsule, brain stem and spinal cord. These are associated with increased tone (spasticity) in the affected muscle groups. The reflexes are exaggerated and clonus (a rhythmical muscle contraction, see p. 136) may be present, but muscle wasting and fasciculations are absent. **Lower motor neuron lesions** result in reduced tone and reflexes, muscle wasting and sometimes fasciculations.

Signs of upper motor neuron lesions

1   Weakness is present in all muscle groups of the lower limb but may be more marked in the flexor muscles. In the upper limb, weakness may be more marked in the extensors. There is very little muscle wasting (unless from disuse).

2 Spasticity: increased tone is present (may be clasp-knife—initial resistance that gives way suddenly) and is often associated with clonus.

3 The reflexes are increased except for the superficial reflexes (e.g. abdominal), which are absent.

4 There is an extensor (Babinski) plantar response (upgoing toe).

Signs of lower motor neuron lesions

1 Weakness may be more obvious distally than proximally, and the flexor and extensor muscles are equally involved. Wasting is a prominent feature.

2 Tone is reduced.

3 The reflexes are reduced and the plantar response is normal or absent.

4 Fasciculation may be present.

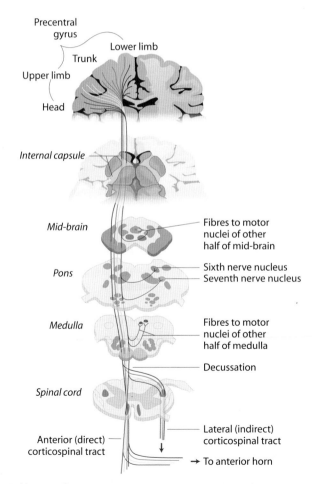

Figure 7.6 Motor pathways

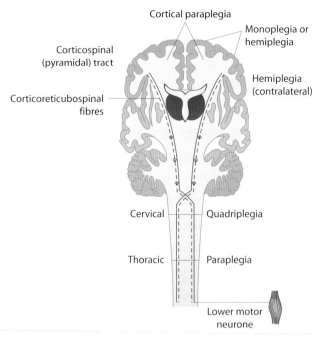

Figure 7.7 Upper and lower motor neuron lesions

Upper limbs

Ask the patient to sit over the side of the bed facing you. Look for abnormal movements.

1. **Tremor.** A tremor is rhythmical oscillation around a joint due to contraction and relaxation of muscles or alternating contraction and relaxation in opposing muscle groups. A normal, fine (>10 cycles/second) tremor is present when muscles attempt to maintain a stationary position against gravity (**physiological tremor**). This is exaggerated with anxiety, alcoholism and thyrotoxicosis, and in patients with a familial tremor. A coarse **resting tremor** occurs in Parkinson's disease: there is repetitive flexion and contraction of the fingers, and abduction and adduction of the thumb (pill rolling tremor) at rest.

2. **Irregular movements. Choreiform** movements are involuntary jerky repetitive movements that may appear to be semi-purposeful; they occur in extrapyramidal disease. Flapping of the tongue (rapid protrusion and retraction with flapping of the tip) is commonly associated. **Athetosis** is a slow writhing movement. The dramatic involuntary swinging movements that characterise **hemiballismus** are rare. **Myoclonic jerks**, on the other hand, are involuntary sudden shock-like muscle contractions that are relatively common.

3. **Pseudoathetosis** (small writhing movements, especially of the fingers) occurs because of proprioceptive (posterior column) loss.

7

Motor system

Examine the motor system systematically every time.

1. Inspect first for **wasting** (both proximal and distal) and **fasciculations**. Don't forget to include the trunk and shoulder girdle in your inspection.
2. Ask the patient to hold out both hands with the arms extended and to close the eyes. Look for **drifting of one or both arms**, which can be due to either (1) upper motor neuron weakness, (2) a cerebellar lesion or (3) proprioceptive loss.
3. Feel the **muscle bulk** of the upper arms and forearms and note any muscle tenderness.
4. Test **tone** at the wrists and elbows by moving the joints passively at varying velocities. Flex and extend the patient's wrists and elbows after asking him or her to relax and not help you. It takes some practice to become familiar with normal muscle tone. Increased tone is easier to detect than decreased tone. Changes in tone are also easier to detect if they are unilateral.
5. Assess **power** (see Fig 7.8) at the shoulders, elbows, wrists and fingers. Remember that right-handed people are slightly stronger on the right side. Power is graded as follows:

   0: complete paralysis
   1: a flicker of contraction
   2: movement is possible where gravity is excluded
   3: movement is possible against gravity but not if any further resistance is added
   4: movement is possible against gravity and some resistance
   5: normal power.

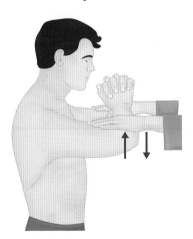

'Stop me pushing your arms down'

(a) Shoulder abduction

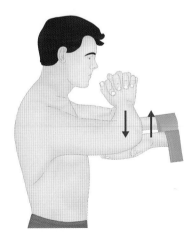

'Stop me pulling your arms up'

(b) Shoulder adduction

Figure 7.8 Testing power in the upper limbs   *continued*

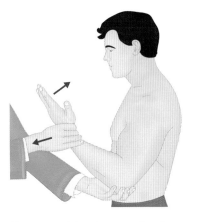

'Stop me straightening your elbow'

(c) Elbow flexion

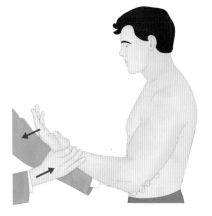

'Stop me bending your elbow'

(d) Elbow extension

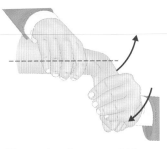

'Stop me bending your wrists'

(e) Wrist flexion

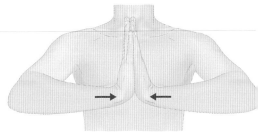

'Put your palms together like this' (demonstrate)

(f) Wrist extension

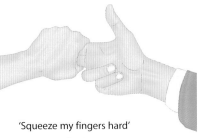

'Squeeze my fingers hard'

(g) Finger flexion

Figure 7.8 Testing power in the upper limbs   *continued*

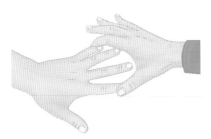 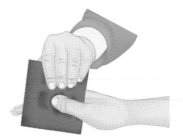

'Stop me bringing your fingers together'   'Hold the paper and stop me pulling it out'

(h) Finger abduction   **(i)** Froment's sign

Figure 7.8 Testing power in the upper limbs *continued*

Shoulder
- **Abduction** (C5, C6 nerve root innervation): the patient should abduct the arms with the elbows flexed and resist your attempt to push them down (see Fig 7.8(a)).
- **Adduction** (C6, C7, C8): the patient should adduct the arms with the elbows flexed and not allow you to separate them (see Fig 7.8(b)).

Elbow
- **Flexion** (C5, C6): the patient should bend the elbow and pull so as not to let you straighten it out (see Fig 7.8(c)).
- **Extension** (C7): the patient should bend the elbow and push so as not to let you bend it (see Fig 7.8(d)).

Wrist
- **Flexion** (C6, C7, C8): the patient should bend the wrist and not allow you to straighten it (see Fig 7.8(e)).
- **Extension** (C7, C8): the patient should extend the wrist and not allow you to bend it (see Fig 7.8(f)).

Fingers
- **Extension** (C7, C8): the patient should straighten the fingers and not allow you to push them down (push with the side of your hand across the patient's metacarpophalangeal joints).
- **Flexion** (C7, C8): the patient squeezes two of your fingers (see Fig 7.8(g)).
- **Abduction** (C8, T1): the patient should spread out the fingers and not allow you to push them together (see Fig 7.8(h)).
- If the patient has a **claw hand** (fixed flexion of the fingers), testing for an **ulnar** or **median** nerve lesion is necessary.
- Look for **wasting of the small muscles of the hand** with deep gutters between the long extensor tendons and hypothenar eminence (ulnar nerve lesion) or thenar eminence (median nerve lesion). Ask the patient to extend both wrists and ask about tingling (**Phalen's sign** from median nerve entrapment in the carpal tunnel syndrome).

- When the patient grasps a piece of paper between the thumb and the lateral aspect of the forefinger, the thumb flexes if an ulnar lesion has caused loss of the adductor of the thumb (**Froment's sign**; see Fig 7.8(i)).
- Ask the patient to place his or her hand flat, with the palm upwards, and then ask the patient to lift the thumb vertically against resistance or to lift the thumb vertically to touch your pen (**pen-touching test** for loss of abductor pollicis brevis—median nerve; see Fig 7.9). This is not possible if there is a median nerve palsy at the wrist or above.

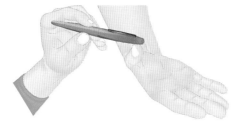

'Lift your thumb to touch my pen, but keep your hand flat on the table'

Figure 7.9 The pen-touching test for loss of abductor pollicis brevis (median nerve)

Reflexes

Examine the reflexes (see Fig 7.10) routinely at the elbow and wrist. Remember that the **reflex arc** consists of afferent and efferent pathways. The afferent pathway is stimulated when a tendon is stretched (e.g. after being struck by a reflex hammer). The afferent pathway synapses in the spinal cord with a motor neuron that fires, stimulating the efferent pathway, and causes contraction of the opposing muscle to release the stretch on the tendon. Interruption of the efferent or afferent limb of the reflex arc prevents contraction and the reflex is absent. Interruption of pathways in the spinal cord above the level of the motor neuron (upper motor neuron lesion) releases this from inhibition and causes exaggerated reflexes (see box on pp. 122–3). Reflexes may be normal, increased, decreased or even absent or delayed (contraction is brisk but return is slow—typical of hypothyroidism).

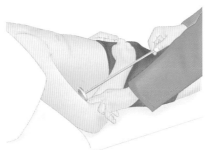

(a) The biceps jerk

Figure 7.10 The biceps, triceps and finger jerks

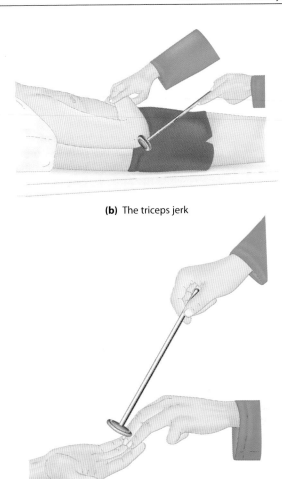

(b) The triceps jerk

(c) The finger jerk

Figure 7.10 The biceps, triceps and finger jerks *continued*

Clonus is rhythmical contraction of the muscle that can continue as long as tension is maintained on the tendon. This occurs with an upper motor neuron lesion. Clonus is not usually tested in the upper limbs.

An idea of the range of normal reflexes can only be obtained by practice. Always compare right with left. Upper limb tendon reflexes are sometimes difficult to elicit in younger patients.

- **Biceps** (C5, C6): place your left forefinger over the biceps tendon and allow the patellar hammer to fall onto it (see Fig 7.10(a)). There is normally a brisk (but not too brisk) contraction of the biceps muscle.
- **Triceps** (C7, C8): support one of the patient's elbows with one hand and tap over the triceps tendon with the hammer (see Fig 7.10(b)). There is normally triceps contraction and extension of the forearm.

- **Brachioradialis** (C5, C6): place a few fingers over the lower end of the radius and strike them. Contraction of the brachioradialis causes flexion of the elbow.
- **Finger** (C8, T1): interlock your hand with the patient's while the patient's hand is resting palm upwards; the tendon hammer is used to strike your hand. Normally, there is slight flexion of all fingers and of the interphalangeal joint of the thumb (see Fig 7.10(c)).
- In patients with suspected upper motor neuron disease, look for **Hoffman's reflex**: the terminal part of the patient's middle finger is flicked downwards between your thumb and finger; it is abnormal if the thumb flexes and adducts while the other fingers flex. The presence of this reflex indicates hyper-reflexia but is not pathognomonic of an upper motor neuron disease.

  The reflexes can be recorded as:

- 0 (absent)
- + (reduced)
- ++ (normal)
- +++ (increased)
- ++++ (exaggerated and with clonus).

Remember motor weakness can be due to an **upper motor neuron lesion** (hyper-reflexia with absence of wasting), a **lower motor neuron lesion** (wasting due to denervation, absent reflexes), **neuromuscular transmission disorders** (fatigue on repeated muscle use) or a **myopathy** (muscle disease usually with wasting but with variable reflexes). If there is evidence of a lower motor neuron lesion, consider anterior horn cell, nerve root or brachial plexus lesions, peripheral nerve lesions or a motor peripheral neuropathy.

Coordination (cerebellar function)

First apply **finger–nose** testing. The patient is asked to touch the tip of your forefinger (the target) with his or her own forefinger and with the arm extended, and then to touch his or her own nose (see Fig 7.11). The movements are alternated rapidly. Cerebellar disease will cause the patient's finger to oscillate and overshoot. It is best to keep the target finger still to obtain a better idea of muscle control.

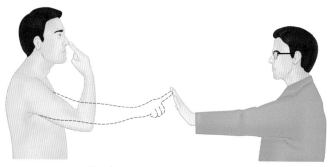

'Touch your nose and then my finger'

Figure 7.11 The cerebellar examination: finger–nose test

Examine for **dysdiadochokinesis**, the inability to perform rapidly alternating movements, such as supinating and pronating the wrists repeatedly (this action appears clumsy in the presence of cerebellar disease).

Next look for **rebound**. Ask the patient to lift both arms quickly from his or her sides then stop halfway. Rebound is present if the patient cannot stop one or both arms.

Sensory system

Examine the sensory system after motor testing because this can be time-consuming. First test the **spinothalamic pathway (pain** and **temperature**; see Fig 7.12). Demonstrate to the patient the sharpness of a new disposable neurology pin or a blunt cannulae that does not break the skin on the anterior chest wall or forehead. Do not use an injection needle, because it is too sharp and can draw blood. Then ask the patient to close his or her eyes and tell you whether the sensation is sharp or dull. Start proximally and test pinprick sensation in each dermatome (see Fig 7.13). As you are assessing, try to fit any sensory loss into **dermatomal** (loss fits into the pattern of one or more dermatomes—cord or nerve root lesion), **peripheral nerve** (pattern specific for the nerve affected, e.g. median or ulnar nerve; see Fig 7.14), **peripheral neuropathy** (affected area is in the shape of a glove) or **hemisensory** (loss involves one side—cortical or cord—distribution). Always compare each side and, as you move up the arms, note the presence of a sensory level (the level of change from abnormal to normal). Tap the pin a number of times in each place to ensure reproducibility.

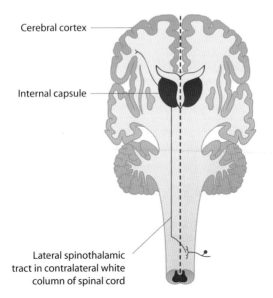

Cerebral cortex

Internal capsule

Lateral spinothalamic tract in contralateral white column of spinal cord

Figure 7.12 Pain and temperature pathways

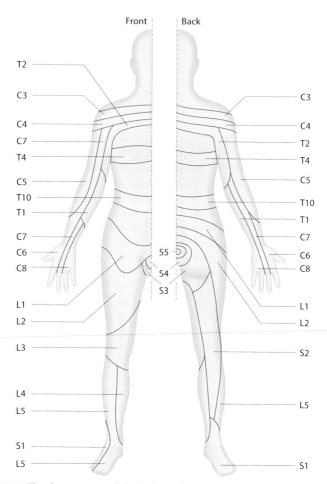

Figure 7.13 The dermatomes of the limbs and trunk

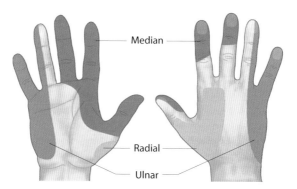

Figure 7.14 Sensory loss of the median and ulnar nerve on the hand

Next test the **posterior column pathway** (**vibration** and **proprioception**; see Fig 7.15). Use a 128 Hz tuning fork to assess vibration sense. Place the vibrating fork on a distal interphalangeal joint when the patient has his or her eyes closed and ask whether the vibrations can be felt. If so, ask the patient to tell you when the vibration ceases and then, after a short wait, stop the fork vibrating. If the patient has deficient sensation, test at the wrist, then the elbow and then at the shoulder to determine the level of the sensory loss.

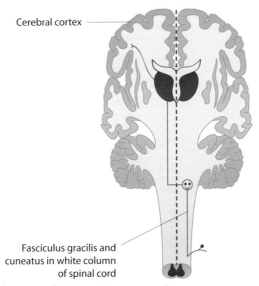

Cerebral cortex

Fasciculus gracilis and cuneatus in white column of spinal cord

Figure 7.15 Vibration and joint position sense pathways

Examine proprioception first with the distal interphalangeal joint of the index finger (see Fig 7.16). When the patient has his or her eyes open, grasp the distal phalanx from the sides and move it up and down to demonstrate. Then ask the patient to close his or her eyes and repeat the manoeuvre, and stop with the phalanx in the up or down position. Repeat this a few times, ending with the phalanx in a different position each time. Normally, movement through even a few degrees is detectable, and the patient can tell whether it is up or down. If there is an abnormality, proceed to test the wrist and elbows similarly to determine the level of the lesion.

Test **light touch** with cottonwool. Touch the skin lightly in each dermatome. Do not wipe the skin as tickle is a spinothalamic sensation.

Test for **cortical sensory abnormalities** if a cortical lesion is suspected after the initial examination. Parietal lobe lesions may cause **sensory inattention**. Here, sensation is normal when one side at a time is tested, but absent on the opposite side to the lesion if both sides are tested together. The patient shuts his or her eyes and both hands are touched. The stimulus is felt only on the normal side. **Astereognosis** also occurs with parietal lesions. This refers to a patient's inability to recognise an object placed in his or her hand.

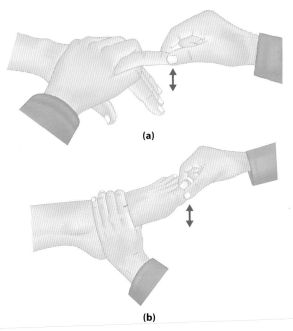

(a)

(b)

'Shut your eyes and tell me whether I have moved your finger (toe) up or down'

Figure 7.16 Testing proprioception: **(a)** finger and **(b)** toe

Lower limbs
Gait

Test the stance and gait first, if possible (see Fig 7.17). Ask the patient to walk normally for a short distance and then to turn around quickly and come back. Then ask the patient to walk heel-to-toe, placing one foot just in front of the other (a test of cerebellar function that has been used by the police to test for alcohol intoxication in less sophisticated times). Next ask the patient to walk on the toes (difficult or impossible with an S1 or tibial nerve lesion) and finally on the heels (difficult or impossible with an L4–5 or peroneal nerve lesion).

Ask the patient to stand with his or her feet together, first with the eyes open and then with them closed. Increased swaying when the eyes are open suggests cerebellar disease. If this occurs only when the eyes are closed (**Romberg's sign**) it suggests proprioceptive loss.

Motor system

1. Lay the patient in bed with the legs entirely exposed. Place a towel over the groin—note whether a urinary catheter is present.
2. Look for **muscle wasting** and **fasciculations**. Note any tremor.
3. Feel the **muscle bulk** of the **quadriceps**, and then run your hand up each shin, feeling for wasting of the **anterior tibial** muscles.

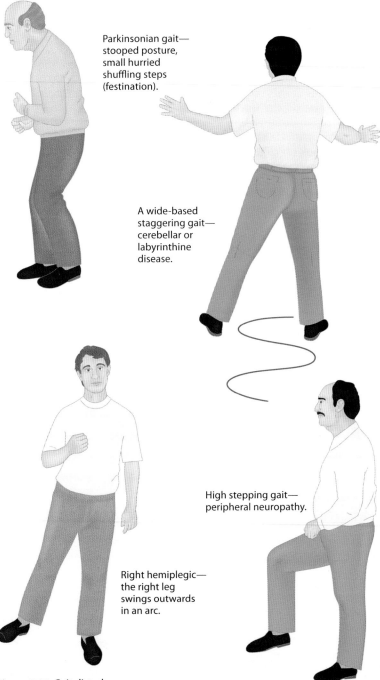

Parkinsonian gait—stooped posture, small hurried shuffling steps (festination).

A wide-based staggering gait—cerebellar or labyrinthine disease.

High stepping gait—peripheral neuropathy.

Right hemiplegic—the right leg swings outwards in an arc.

Figure 7.17 Gait disturbances

4. Test **tone** at the knees and ankles. The patient lies supine and is asked to relax and not oppose or assist your movement of the limbs. Place your hand under the patient's knee and lift the knee quickly so that it flexes and extends. Then grasp the foot and flex and extend it repeatedly. With practice, normal and abnormal muscle resistance to these movements will be appreciated.

5. Test **clonus** at this time. Push the lower end of the quadriceps sharply down towards the knee. Sustained rhythmical contractions of the quadriceps indicate an upper motor neuron lesion. Also test the ankle by sharply dorsiflexing the foot with the knee bent and the thigh externally rotated; look for clonus of the calf muscles.

6. Assess **power** next at the hips, knees and ankles (see Fig 7.18). This should again be graded from 0 to 5 (see p. 125).

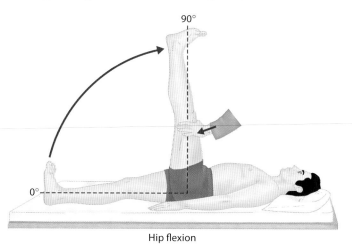

'Stop me pushing your leg down'
(a) Hip flexion

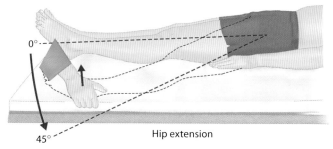

'Push your heel into the bed and stop me lifting it up'
(b) Hip extension

Figure 7.18 Testing power in the lower limbs

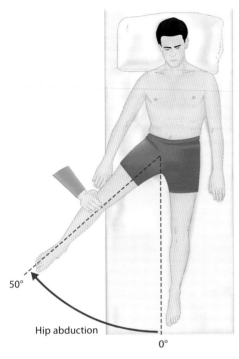

50°

Hip abduction

0°

'Stop me pushing your leg inwards'

(c) Hip abduction

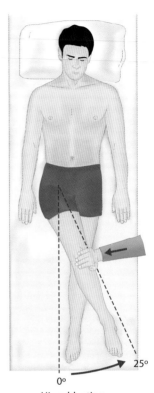

25°

0°

Hip adduction

'Push your leg sideways
against my hand'

(d) Hip adduction

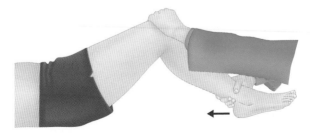

'Bend your leg and stop me straightening it'

(e) Knee flexion

Figure 7.18 Testing power in the lower limbs   *continued*

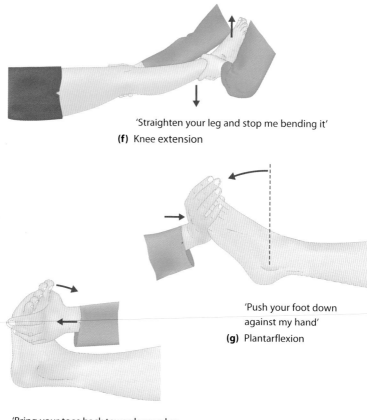

'Straighten your leg and stop me bending it'
(f) Knee extension

'Push your foot down
against my hand'
(g) Plantarflexion

'Bring your toes back towards your leg
and stop me pushing them down'
(h) Dorsiflexion (ankle)

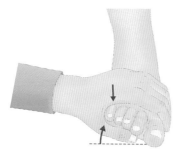

'Twist your foot out and
stop me straightening it'
(i) Eversion

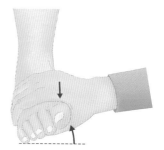

'Twist your foot in and
stop me straightening it'
(j) Inversion

Figure 7.18 Testing power in the lower limbs *continued*

Hip

- **Flexion** (L2, L3 innervation): ask the patient to lift up the straight leg and not to let you push it down (having placed your hand above the knee; see Fig 7.18(a)).
- **Extension** (S1): ask the patient to keep the leg down and not to let you pull it up from underneath the calf or ankle (see Fig 7.18(b)).
- **Abduction** (L5): ask the patient to abduct the leg and not to let you push it in (see Fig 7.18(c)).
- **Adduction** (L2, L3): ask the patient to keep the leg adducted and not to let you push it out (see Fig 7.18(d)).

Knee

- **Flexion** (L5, S1): ask the patient to bend the knee and not to let you straighten it (see Fig 7.18(e)).
- **Extension** (L3, L4): with the knee slightly bent, ask the patient to straighten the knee and not to let you bend it (see Fig 7.18(f)).

Ankle

- **Plantarflexion** (S1, S2): ask the patient to push the foot down and not to let you push it up (see Fig 7.18(g)).
- **Dorsiflexion** (L4, L5): ask the patient to bring the foot up and not to let you push it down (see Fig 7.18(h)).
- **Eversion** (L5): ask the patient to evert the foot against resistance (see Fig 7.18(i)).
- **Inversion** (L5, S1): with the foot in complete plantarflexion, ask the patient to invert the foot against resistance (see Fig 7.18(j)).

Reflexes

Examine the **reflexes** (see Fig 7.19).

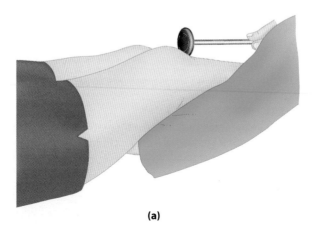

(a)

Figure 7.19 (a) The knee jerk   *continued*

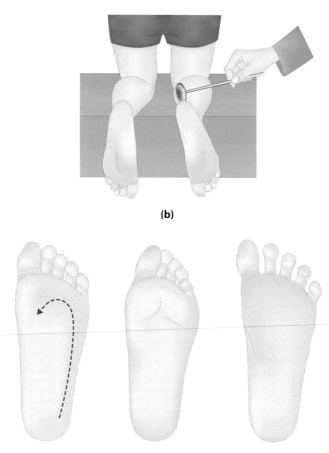

(b)

'I'm going to scratch the bottom of your foot'

(c) Line of stroke   PLANTAR REFLEX   EXTENSOR RESPONSE
                            Toes plantarflex   (abnormal) Fanning
                                                  and dorsiflexion of toes

Figure 7.19 (b) The ankle jerk **(c)** The plantarflexes *continued*

Knee (L3, L4)
Allow the patellar hammer to fall elegantly onto the infrapatellar tendon while the patient's knee is supported by the examiner's arm (see Fig 7.19(a)). Watch for contraction of the quadriceps.

Ankle (S1, S2)
The patient's foot is in the mid-position at the ankle, the knee is bent and the thigh is externally rotated on the bed. The patellar hammer is allowed to fall onto the patellar (Achilles) tendon (see Fig 7.19(b)). Plantar flexion of the foot will normally occur. The reflex can also be elicited by having the patient kneel and directly tapping the tendon.

Plantar response (L5, S1, S2)

A key or similar object is run slowly along the lateral aspect of the patient's sole (see Fig 7.19(c)). The normal response is flexion of the great toe. Upper motor neuron lesions result in extension (dorsiflexion) of the great toe and fanning of the other toes. This is described as an upgoing (extensor) plantar response or a **Babinski sign**. This sign is normal in infants.

Coordination (cerebellar function)

Perform:

1. the **heel–shin** test (the patient runs the heel of one foot up and down the shin of the other leg as rapidly and accurately as possible, while you look for wobbling or the heel falling off; see Fig 7.20)
2. the **toe–finger** test (the patient brings the toe up to touch your forefinger with the knee bent, while you look for tremor and overshooting)
3. **tapping of the feet** (the patient taps the sole of the foot on your hand, while you look for clumsy or slow movements—**dysdiadochokinesis**).

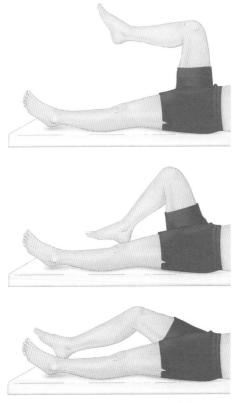

'Lift your right leg up, place your heel on your left knee and then run it quickly down your shin'

Figure 7.20 Test coordination: heel–shin test

Sensory system

Test **pain** (pinprick), then **vibration** and **proprioception**, and then **light touch** (as described for the upper limbs and in each dermatome on both sides) (see Fig 7.14). If sensory loss involves the entire leg or both legs, attempt to establish where normal sensation begins on the trunk or chest (the sensory level).

Test the **abdominal reflexes**. Stroke the skin of the lower abdominal wall with a sharpish object such as a key in each quadrant, first on one side and then on the other. Brisk contraction of the underlying muscles normally occurs. Test the upper and lower quadrants on both sides. Absent reflexes may be a result of an upper motor neuron lesion, but lax abdominal muscles or previous surgery that has cut the superficial abdominal nerves may also cause reflex loss.

Examine sensation in the **saddle region** (perineum and medial aspects of the upper thighs) region. Test the **anal reflex** (S2, S3, S4); there is normally contraction of the external sphincter in response to scratching of the perianal skin.

The spine

Examine the **back**. Look for deformity, scars and neurofibromas. Palpate for tenderness over the vertebral bodies and auscultate for bruits. Any of these may indicate spinal cord abnormalities.

Perform the **straight leg raising test**. Lay the patient flat and slowly flex the hip while keeping the knee fully extended. Tell the patient to advise you as soon as there is pain and where it occurs (a disc compression of the lumbar or sacral roots will limit leg raising, because of pain in the ipsilateral leg that will be increased by foot dorsiflexion). With more severe nerve root irritation the pain will be felt in the other lower limb as well (crossed straight leg raising sign). Test the upper lumbar roots by laying the patient prone and extending the hip (while the knee is flexed to 90°) (see **femoral nerve stretch test**, p. 178).

The neurological history and examination OSCE: hints panel

1 This man has had problems with confusion. Please examine him.

(a) General inspection:* stand back and look for signs of dehydration, malnutrition or cyanosis or recent evidence of trauma.

(b) Test orientation for time, place and person.

(c) Perform a mini-mental state examination.

(d) Measure his pulse and blood pressure (hypertensive encephalopathy). Look for signs of cardiac failure.

(e) Look for signs of alcoholism and liver failure.

(f) Take his temperature and look for any obvious focus of infection.

(g) Ask to test his urine and blood sugar (hypoglycaemia or diabetes mellitus).

(h) Ask to review his medication chart.

(i) Synthesise and present your findings.
   * Delirium or confusion is usually a multifactorial condition.

2 Please assess this woman's gait. She has had difficulty walking.

(a) See whether it is possible for the patient to expose her legs to the mid-thigh. Look for joint deformity.

(b) Ask the patient whether she can walk.

(c) Ask her to walk backwards and forwards; look at the gait for any characteristic abnormality.

(d) If she seems steady enough, ask her to walk heel-to-toe. Demonstrate this for her.

(e) Test Romberg's sign.

(f) Ask her to squat and stand (tests proximal muscle strength).

(g) Ask her to stand on her toes and then on her heels (tests more distal power).

(h) If indicated, ask her to lie down and test the lower limbs neurologically.

(i) Synthesise and present your findings.

3 This man has felt unsteady and clumsy. Please examine his coordination.

(a) Examine for nystagmus (typically jerky, with an increased amplitude on looking to the side of a cerebellar lesion).

(b) Test for dysarthria (e.g. say 'British constitution'). Note any jerky, loud explosive cerebellar type speech.

(c) Test arm drift (hypotonia, in cerebellar disease on the same side as the lesion).

(d) Assess the finger–nose test (for intention tremor and past pointing) and rapidly alternating movements (dysdiadokinesis). Then test rebound.

(e) Assess leg tone, then the heel–skin test, intention tremor (big toe to your finger) and heel tapping on the other shin.

(f) Ask the patient to fold his arms and sit up (truncal ataxia).

(g) Assess gait (staggering towards the side of the cerebellar lesion).

(h) Examine the cranial nerves (e.g. fifth, seventh and eighth lesions on one side from a cerebellopontine angle tumour).

(i) Auscultate over the skull for a cerebellar bruit.

(j) Auscultate for carotid bruits.

(k) Synthesise and present your findings.

The neurological examination
hints for success

1   A careful neurological history should direct the neurological examination to the most relevant areas. Symptoms may occur before signs can be detected, but in the absence of symptoms any signs are less likely to be important.

2   The methodical approach that characterises the skilled neurological examination helps define the anatomical site of the abnormality.

3   A careful neurological examination will usually enable you to develop a sensible differential diagnosis.

4   Note the distribution of signs and look particularly for asymmetrical abnormalities.

5   Normal people may have no gag or abdominal reflexes.

6   Absent tendon reflexes usually indicate an abnormality in the sensory or motor system.

7   An extensor plantar reflex that is reproducible is never normal (except in infants).

8   Hepatitis B and C virus, and HIV, have been isolated from needles used to test pin-prick sensation. Disposable needles or blunt cannulae should always be used.

chapter 8

The eyes, ears, nose and throat

Out vile jelly! Where is thy lustre now?

William Shakespeare, *King Lear* (1604–5)

The examination of the eyes, ears, nose and throat is usually directed by the history. These small parts of the body may provide vital diagnostic clues in neurological or systemic disease.

The eyes

Examination anatomy

The structure of the eye is shown in Figure 8.1. Much of this structure can be examined as outlined below. Figure 8.2 shows the muscles responsible for eye movements and their innervation.

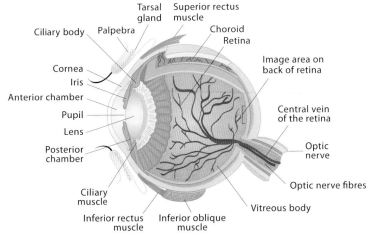

Figure 8.1 The structure of the eye

Examination method

Sit the patient at the edge of the bed facing you. Standing well back from the patient, inspect for:

1. **ptosis** (drooping of one or both upper eyelids)
2. **colour of the sclerae:**
   - **yellow** (deposits of bilirubin in jaundice)
   - **blue** (which may be due to osteogenesis imperfecta, because the thin sclerae allow the choroidal pigment to show through; blue sclerae can also occur in families without osteogenesis imperfecta)
   - **red (iritis**, which causes central inflammation; or **conjunctivitis**, which causes more peripheral inflammation often with pus; or **subconjunctival haemorrhage** as a result of trauma)
   - **scleral pallor**, which occurs in anaemia. Pull down the lower lid and look for the normal contrast between the pearly white posterior conjunctiva and the red anterior part. Loss of this contrast is a reliable sign of anaemia.

Look from behind and above the patient for **exophthalmos**, which is prominence of the eyes. If there is actual protrusion of the eyes from the orbits, this is called **proptosis**. This is best detected by looking at the eyes from above the forehead; protrusion beyond the supraorbital ridge is abnormal. If exophthalmos is present, examine specifically for thyroid eye disease (p. 115): lid lag (the patient follows your finger as it descends—the upper lid lags behind the pupil), chemosis (oedema of the bulbar conjunctiva), corneal ulceration and ophthalmoplegia (weakness of upward gaze; see Ch 7). A drop of sterile fluorescein will stain **corneal ulcers**.

Proceed then as for the cranial nerve examination (p. 117)—that is, testing visual acuity, visual fields (see Fig 7.4) and pupillary responses to light and accommodation. Look for an **afferent pupillary defect** (or Marcus Gunn sign). Move the torch in an arc from pupil to pupil—an abnormal pupil will paradoxically dilate when the torch is moved to the abnormal eye, as occurs in optic atrophy.

Test the **eye movements** (see Fig 8.2). Look also for fatigability of eye muscles by asking the patient to look up at a hat pin or finger for about half a minute. In myasthenia gravis the muscles tire and the eyelids begin to droop.

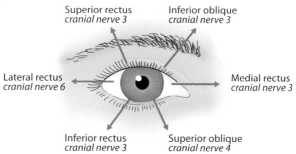

Superior rectus
cranial nerve 3

Inferior oblique
cranial nerve 3

Lateral rectus
cranial nerve 6

Medial rectus
cranial nerve 3

Inferior rectus
cranial nerve 3

Superior oblique
cranial nerve 4

Figure 8.2 Eye movements, muscles and innervation (right eye)

Test **colour vision** if acuity is not poor. You can use Ishihara test plates (where coloured spots form numbers). Red desaturation (impaired ability to see red objects) can occur with optic nerve disease. Red–green colour blindness affects 7% of males (X-linked recessive).

Test the **corneal reflex** (p. 120).

Consider the possibility that the patient may have a glass eye. This should be suspected if visual acuity is zero in one eye and no pupillary reaction is apparent. Attempts to examine and interpret the fundus of a glass eye will amuse the patient but are always unsuccessful.

Horner's syndrome

Interruption of the sympathetic innervation of the eye at any point results in **Horner's syndrome**. This causes **partial ptosis** (as sympathetic fibres supply the smooth muscle of both eyelids) and a **constricted pupil** (because of an unbalanced parasympathetic action), which reacts normally to light. There may be reduced sweating on the forehead on the affected side (anhydrosis).

Note that perceptible anisocoria (inequality of the diameters of the pupils) is found in 20% of normal people. Its presence should not always cause alarm. Remember also that elderly people quite often have imperceptible pupillary light reactions.

Ophthalmoscopy

Successful ophthalmoscopy requires considerable practice. It is important that it be performed in reduced ambient lighting so that the patient's pupils are at least partly dilated and you are not distracted. It can be easier to perform the examination, especially of the fundi, through the patient's spectacles. Otherwise, the patient's refractive error should be corrected by use of the appropriate ophthalmoscope lens. The patient should be asked to stare at a point on the opposite wall or on the ceiling and to ignore the light of the ophthalmoscope. Patients will often attempt to focus on the ophthalmoscope light and should be asked not to do this initially.

Begin by examining the **cornea**. Use your right eye to examine the patient's right eye, and vice versa. Turn the ophthalmoscope lens to +20 and examine the cornea from about 20 cm away from the patient. Look particularly for corneal ulceration. Turn the lens gradually down to 0 while moving closer to the patient. Structures, including the **lens, humour** and then the retina at increasing distance into the eye, will swim into focus.

Examine the **retinas**. Focus on one of the retinal arteries and follow it into the optic disc. The **normal optic disc** is round and paler than the surrounding retina. The margin of the disc is usually sharply outlined but will appear blurred if there is papilloedema or papillitis, or pale if there is optic atrophy. Inspect the rest of the retina and especially look for the retinal changes of diabetes mellitus or hypertension.

There are two main types of retinal change in **diabetes mellitus**: non-proliferative and proliferative. Non-proliferative changes include: (1) two types of haemorrhages—**dot haemorrhages**, which occur in the inner retinal layers, and **blot haemorrhages**, which are larger and occur more superficially in the nerve fibre layer; (2) **microaneurysms** (tiny bulges in the vessel wall), which are due to vessel wall damage; and (3) two types of exudates—**hard exudates**, which have straight edges and are due to leakage of protein from damaged arteriolar walls, and **soft exudates** (cottonwool spots), which have a fluffy appearance and are due to microinfarcts. Proliferative changes include new vessel formation, which can lead to retinal detachment or vitreous haemorrhage.

Hypertensive changes can be classified from grades 1 to 4:

- **grade 1:** 'silver wiring' of the arteries only (sclerosis of the vessel wall reduces its transparency so that the central light streak becomes broader and shinier)
- **grade 2:** silver wiring of arteries plus arteriovenous nipping or nicking (indentation or deflection of the veins where they are crossed by the arteries)
- **grade 3:** grade 2 plus haemorrhages (flame-shaped) and exudates (soft—cottonwool spots due to ischaemia, or hard—lipid residues from leaking vessels)
- **grade 4:** grade 3 changes plus papilloedema.

It is important to describe the changes present rather than just give a grade.

Inspect carefully for **central retinal artery occlusion** where the whole fundus appears milky-white because of retinal oedema, and the arteries become greatly reduced in diameter.

Central retinal vein thrombosis causes tortuous retinal veins and haemorrhages scattered over the whole retina, particularly occurring alongside the veins.

Retinitis pigmentosa causes a scattering of black pigment in a criss-cross pattern. This will be missed if the periphery of the retina is not examined.

Finally, ask the patient to look directly at the light. This allows you to locate and inspect the **macula** (an oval, yellow spot near the centre of the retina that is important for central vision).

The ears
Examination anatomy
The pinna, external auditory canal and ear drum (see Fig 8.3) are easily assessed with simple equipment. Tests of hearing can also provide information about the severity and anatomical site of hearing loss.

Examination method
Ear examination consists of **inspection** and **palpation**, **auriscopic examination** and **testing hearing**.

Inspect the position of the **pinna** and note its size and shape. Note any scars or swelling around the ears. Look for an obvious accessory auricle (separate piece of cartilage away from the pinna), cauliflower ears (haematomas from recurrent trauma, which fill in the hollows of the ear) and bat ears (protrusion of the ears from the side of the head).

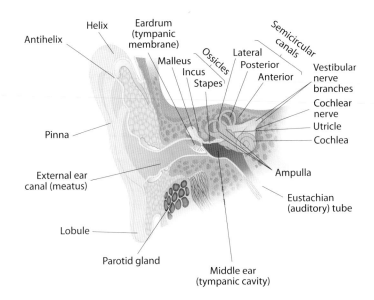

Figure 8.3 Cross-sectional anatomy of the ear showing the pinna, external auditory canal, middle and inner ear

Look for signs of inflammation, including gouty tophi (nodular, firm, pale and non-tender chalky depositions of urate in the cartilage of the ear, specific but not sensitive for gout). Then look for any obvious ear *discharge.*

Palpate the pinna for swelling or nodules. Pull down the pinna gently; infection of the external canal often causes tenderness of the pinna.

Auriscopic examination of the ears requires use of an earpiece that fits comfortably in the ear canal to allow inspection of the ear canal and tympanic membrane. This examination is essential if there is a history of recent deafness or a painful ear. Examination is also necessary in the patient who has had a head injury. Always examine both ears!

The correct technique is as follows (see Fig 8.4). Ask the patient to turn his or her head slightly to the side, then pull the pinna up, out and back to straighten the ear canal and provide optimal vision. Stretch out the fingers of the hand holding the auriscope to touch the patient's cheek, to steady the instrument and prevent sudden movements of the patient's head. When examining the patient's right ear, the auriscope is preferably held in a *downward position* with the right hand, while using the left hand to pull the pinna. An alternative position involves holding the auriscope upwards, but there is a risk that if the patient moves suddenly injury is more likely to occur.

Look at the **external canal** for any evidence of inflammation (e.g. redness or swelling) or discharge. There should be no tenderness unless there is inflammation. Ear **wax** is white or yellowish, and translucent and shiny; it may obscure the view of the tympanic membrane. Blood or cerebrospinal

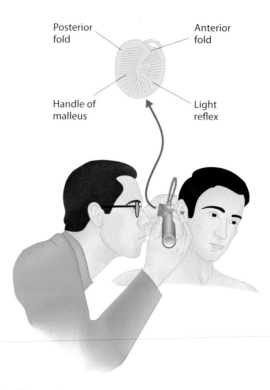

Posterior fold

Anterior fold

Handle of malleus

Light reflex

Figure 8.4 Use of the auriscope

fluid (watery, clear fluid) may be seen in the canal if there is a fracture at the base of the skull. In patients with herpes zoster, there may be vesicles (fluid-filled blisters) on the posterior wall around the external auditory meatus.

Inspect the **tympanic membrane** (eardrum) by introducing the speculum further into the canal in a forward but downward direction. The normal tympanic membrane is greyish and reflects light from the centre at approximately 5 or 7 o'clock. Note the colour, transparency and any evidence of dilated blood vessels. Look for bulging or retraction of the tympanic membrane. Bulging can suggest underlying fluid or pus in the middle ear. Perforation of the tympanic membrane should be noted.

If a middle ear infection is suspected, **pneumatic auriscopy** can be useful. Use a speculum large enough to occlude the external canal snugly. Attach a rubber squeeze bulb to the auriscope. When the bulb is squeezed gently, air pressure in the canal is increased and the tympanic membrane should move promptly inward. Absence of, or a decrease in, movement is a sign of fluid in the middle ear.

To **test hearing**, whisper numbers 60 cm away from one of the patient's ears while the other ear is distracted by movement of your finger in the auditory canal. Then repeat the process with the other ear. With practice the normal range of hearing is appreciated. Then perform Rinné's and Weber's tests:

1. **Rinné's test**: place a vibrating 256 Hz tuning fork on the mastoid process. When the sound is no longer heard move the fork close to the auditory meatus where, if air conduction is, as is normal, better than bone conduction, it will again be audible.
2. **Weber's test:** place a vibrating 256 Hz fork at the centre of the patient's forehead. Nerve deafness causes the sound to be heard better in the normal ear, but with conduction deafness the opposite occurs.

The nose
Examination method

Nose examination consists of **inspection, palpation** and **testing sense of smell**.

Look at the skin. Note any nasal deviation (best seen from behind the patient looking down). Note any periorbital swelling (e.g. from sinusitis). Inspect the nares by pressing the tip of the nose upwards with your thumb.

Palpate the nasal bones. Then feel for facial swelling or signs of inflammation. Block each nostril to assess any obstruction by asking the patient to inhale.

If there is a history of anosmia (loss of smell), test smell (cranial nerve I; p. 117).

The throat
Examination anatomy

See Figure 8.5.

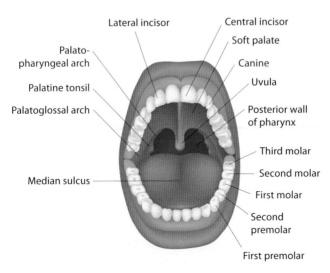

Figure 8.5 The mouth and throat

Examination method

Throat examination consists of **inspection** and **palpation**.

Look in turn at the lips, buccal mucosa, gums, palate and teeth. Note any signs of inflammation (e.g. redness, swelling). Inspect the tongue first in the mouth, then ask the patient to poke it out, and then ask the patient to touch it to the roof of the mouth (to look at the floor of the mouth).

Ask the patient to say 'Aaah', then inspect the oropharynx and uvula (you often need to press a tongue depressor on the posterior tongue to see properly). Inspect the tonsils (note the size, shape, colour, discharge or membrane—they involute in adults and may not be seen).

Palpate the tongue for lumps (wear gloves).

Palpate the salivary glands (p. 104). Finally, examine the cervical lymph nodes (p. 102).

The eyes, ears, nose and throat OSCE: hints panel

1 **Examine this patient's sclerae and conjunctivae.**

   (a) Stand back to look. This is probably a spot diagnosis.

   (b) Look for scleral icterus. Proceed accordingly if present to examine for signs of chronic liver disease.

   (c) Note the distribution of any redness (e.g. single red eye in iritis). Decide whether conjunctival injection is central (iritis) or spares the central region (conjunctivitis).

   (d) If there is conjunctival injection, ask for gloves before pulling the lower lid down. Note any ocular discharge (conjunctivitis).

   (e) If there is pallor, pull down the lower lid and compare the pearly white posterior part of the conjunctiva with the red anterior part.

   (f) If there is chemosis, look for proptosis and other signs of thyrotoxicosis.

   (g) Look at the iris (haziness indicates oedema or inflammation).

   (h) Look at and test the pupils (e.g. small irregular pupil in iritis; dilated, oval, poorly reactive pupil in acute glaucoma).

   (i) Assess eye movements (painful in scleritis).

   (j) Perform fundoscopy.

   (k) Look for systemic evidence of vasculitis (e.g. urinalysis).

   (l) Synthesise and present your findings.

2 **Look in this patient's fundi.**

   (a) The pupils will probably have been dilated.

   (b) Use the ophthalmoscope in the approved manner.

   (c) Look particularly for changes of hypertension or diabetes.

   (d) Synthesise and present your findings.

3 **This woman has experienced sudden loss of vision in one eye. Please examine her.**

   (a) Test *each* eye for visual acuity, and fully assess the visual fields.

   (b) Assess each pupil's reaction to light and accommodation, and for an afferent pupillary defect (optic nerve damage).

(c) Test eye movements and ask about any pain on movement (optic neuritis).

(d) Examine the fundi. Note whether the disc is swollen and is abnormally pink or white (ischaemic optic neuropathy). Note any retinal fundal pallor (arterial occlusion), haemorrhages (venous occlusion) or an obvious embolus (at an arterial bifurcation).

(e) Test colour vision if red–green test plates are available (for optic nerve damage).

(f) Auscultate for a carotid bruit (stenosis).

(g) Take her pulse (atrial fibrillation) and blood pressure (hypertension).

(h) Ask whether you may test the patient's urine for blood or protein (vasculitis).

(i) Synthesise and present your findings.

4 This man complains of a sore ear. Examine his auditory canal and ear drum.

(a) Note whether he looks unwell or feverish.

(b) Look at the pinna and external auditory meatus for gouty tophi, dermatitis, cellulitis, signs of trauma (e.g. haematoma), scars (e.g. surgery) and discharge. Look at *both* ears.

(c) Ask the patient whether the ear is painful before using the auriscope to examine the canal and drum.

(d) Look for erythema or blisters in the canal, and for wax, pus or discharge from the drum.

(e) Inspect the tympanic membrane (ear drum) for perforation, grommets (tympanostomy tubes) or loss of the normal shiny appearance.

(f) Test hearing, and perform Rinné's and Weber's tests.

(g) Palpate the temporomandibular joint for tenderness and crepitus (referred pain).

(h) Examine the throat for inflammation (referred pain).

(i) Synthesise and present your findings.

5 This patient complains of recurrent sore throat. Please examine her.

(a) Put on gloves. Remove dentures if the patient wears them. Note any drooling or flushing, or whether she appears ill.

(b) Take a torch and ask the patient to open wide.

(c) Inspect her mouth and pharynx using a tongue depressor. Note tonsillar enlargement and any erythema or other signs of inflammation.

(d) Note whether the patient cannot open her mouth fully (trismus).

(e) Feel the oral cavity and tongue gently with a gloved finger.

(f) Palpate the cervical nodes carefully.

(g) Take her temperature (fever).

(h) Ask to refer for an examination of the nostrils with an auriscope (e.g. rhinitis) and indirect laryngoscopy, if indicated. Other tests may include a throat swab (bacterial tonsillitis) and monospot test (glandular fever).

(i) Synthesise and present your findings.

The eyes, ears, nose and throat   hints for success

1 Important local and systemic disease can be missed unless the eyes are examined as part of a general medical examination.
2 Accurate fundoscopy with the ophthalmoscope requires practice. Dilating the patient's pupils may be necessary to obtain an adequate view.
3 Subtle eye signs, such as Horner's syndrome, will be missed unless time is taken to stand back and compare the two sides.
4 Complete examination of the mouth and throat includes palpating the draining lymph nodes (cervical nodes).

chapter **9**

The thyroid and endocrine system

The thyroid gland ... is that organ which when enlarged by disease gives rise to 'Derbyshire neck' or goitre.

Thomas Huxley (1825–1895)

The thyroid

Presenting symptoms

The thyroid is a small gland that is usually unobtrusive but that exerts a powerful influence on all parts of the body. Under- or overactivity produces characteristic symptoms and signs:

- **Thyrotoxicosis** (excess thyroid hormone production) can cause a preference for cooler weather, weight loss, increased appetite (polyphagia), palpitations (sinus tachycardia or atrial fibrillation), increased sweating, nervousness, irritability, diarrhoea, amenorrhoea, muscle weakness and exertional dyspnoea.
- **Hypothyroidism** (myxoedema—decreased thyroid hormone production) can result in a preference for warmer weather, weight gain, lethargy, swelling of eyelids (oedema), hoarse voice, constipation and coarse dry skin.

The history

Find out about previous surgery (e.g. thyroidectomy) and about other treatments for thyroid disease, such as radioiodine, anti-thyroid drugs or thyroid replacement treatment.

Many endocrine conditions are chronic and their effect on a patient's ability to work and look after him or herself must be assessed.

There may be a history in the family of thyroid conditions. Find out where the patient grew up (there are areas of endemic goitre caused by iodine deficiency).

Examination anatomy

The word thyroid comes from the Greek *thyreoeides*, meaning a shield. It sits like a shield in the front of the neck (see Fig 9.1). Its two lobes are connected by an isthmus, which lies just below the larynx. It may be palpable in normal thin people.

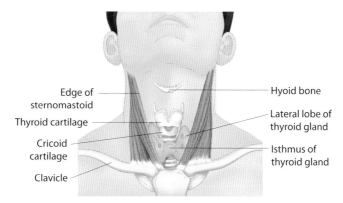

Edge of sternomastoid

Thyroid cartilage

Cricoid cartilage

Clavicle

Hyoid bone

Lateral lobe of thyroid gland

Isthmus of thyroid gland

Figure 9.1 Surface anatomy of the neck and thyroid

Examination of the thyroid

The thyroid should be examined first by **inspection**, followed by **palpation**, **percussion** and **auscultation**.

Inspection

Sometimes the isthmus of the normal thyroid is visible as a diffuse central swelling in the neck. Enlargement of the gland, called a **goitre** (from the Latin *guttur*, meaning throat), should be apparent on inspection. Look at the front and sides of the neck and decide whether there is localised or general swelling of the gland.

Then ask the patient to **swallow a sip of water** while you watch the swelling. Only a goitre or a **thyroglossal cyst** will rise during swallowing, because of their attachment to the larynx. Ask the patient to **stick out his or her tongue**: a thyroglossal cyst will move up, but a goitre will not.

Inspect the skin of the neck for scars and look for prominent veins (suggesting thoracic inlet obstruction caused by a retrosternal thyroid mass).

Palpation

Systematically feel both lobes of the gland and its isthmus from behind the patient using the tips of the fingers (see Fig 9.2). Note the size, shape, consistency, symmetry, tenderness and mobility of the gland and the presence of a thrill. Decide whether the lower limit of the gland is palpable. Ask the patient to swallow and feel for the swelling to rise. Feel next for the cervical lymph nodes (p. 102).

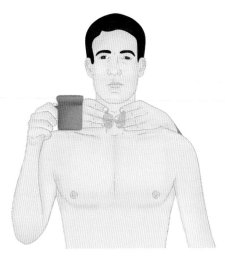

Figure 9.2 Examination of the thyroid

Percussion

Percuss over the upper sternum. Dullness may indicate a retrosternal goitre. Test for **Pemberton's sign**. Ask the patient to lift up both arms as high as possible. In thoracic inlet obstruction (e.g. by a retrosternal goitre), the patient's face will turn red, cyanosis will occur, the neck veins will swell and stridor (harsh inspiration caused by a partly occluded upper airway) may occur.

Auscultation

Auscultate over the gland. A soft bruit may be audible when an overactive gland is very vascular. Listen to the patient's breathing for stridor. If there is a goitre, apply mild compression to the lateral lobes and listen again for stridor.

Thyrotoxicosis

Examine a suspected case of thyrotoxicosis as follows.
1. Look for signs of weight loss, anxiety and the frightened facies of the thyrotoxic (see Fig 9.3).

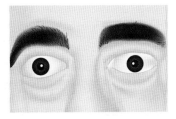

Figure 9.3 Thyrotoxicosis: thyroid stare and exophthalmos

2. Ask the patient to put out his or her arms and look for a **fine tremor**.
3. Look at the patient's nails for **onycholysis** (Plummer's nails—separation of the distal nail from the nail bed) and for thyroid acropachy (clubbing).
4. Inspect for **palmar erythema** (a red appearance of the outer parts of the palms) and feel the palms for warmth and sweatiness (from sympathetic overactivity).
5. Take the patient's **pulse**. Note the presence of sinus tachycardia or atrial fibrillation. The pulse may also have a collapsing character due to a high cardiac output.
6. Test for **proximal myopathy** (weakness of the muscles at the shoulders and hips) and tap the arm reflexes for abnormal briskness, especially in the relaxation phase.
7. Examine the **eyes**. Look for **exophthalmos** (protrusion of the eyeball out of the orbit). Then examine for **lid retraction**, which is suggested by a widened palpebral fissure. Test for **lid lag** by watching for lagging of the descent of the upper lid as the patient follows your finger while you move it at moderate speed from the upper to the lower part of the visual field. Then stand behind the patient and look over the forehead to assess for the degree of **proptosis**, which is actual protrusion of the globes from the orbits.
   Next look for:
   • chemosis (oedema of the conjunctivae)
   • conjunctivitis (inflammation of the conjunctivae)
   • corneal ulceration (it may be necessary to stain the cornea with fluorescein)
   • optic atrophy (rare—pallor of the optic disc when examined with the ophthalmoscope, and due to ischaemia of the retina from stretching in exophthalmos)
   • ophthalmoplegia (upward gaze tends to be lost first, and later convergence is weakened).
8. Examine for thyroid enlargement. A thrill may be present over the gland on palpation. Listen over the gland for a bruit.
9. Examine the **heart** for systolic flow murmurs and for signs of cardiac failure (see Ch 4).
10. Look for **pretibial myxoedema** (bilateral firm and elevated nodules and plaques on the shins, which may be pink or brown).
11. Test for **hyper-reflexia** in the legs.

Hypothyroidism
Examine the patient with suspected hypothyroidism as follows.
1. A variable number of the following signs may be present. Look for signs of obvious mental and physical **sluggishness**. Note peripheral cyanosis, a cool and dry skin and the yellow skin discolouration of hypercarotenaemia (a result of reduced metabolism of carotene).
2. Take the patient's **pulse**, which may be of small volume and slow.
3. Test for **median nerve entrapment** (carpal tunnel syndrome). **Phalen's sign** (tingling in the median nerve distribution during prolonged

extension of the wrist) is more accurate than Tinel's sign (tapping over the flexor retinaculum causing paraesthesia in the tendon sheath when the test is positive).

4. Look at the patient's **face**. The skin, but not the sclera, may appear yellow due to hypercarotenaemia. The skin may be generally thickened, and **alopecia** (loss of hair) may be present, as may **vitiligo** (an associated autoimmune disease).
5. Inspect the **eyes** for periorbital oedema and xanthelasma and note loss or thinning of the outer third of the eyebrows.
6. Ask the patient to speak, and listen for **coarse, croaking, slow speech**.
7. Test for a **'hung up' ankle reflex** with the patient kneeling on a chair (the foot plantarflexes normally when the Achilles tendon is tapped, but then dorsiflexes much more slowly).

Diabetes mellitus

In patients with diabetes mellitus, you need to assess carefully for complications that are often multi-system. One approach is as follows:

1. **General inspection.** Look for signs of dehydration. Weigh the patient (obesity). Note the patient's mental state (coma can occur). There may be signs of Cushing's syndrome or acromegaly (secondary causes of diabetes mellitus).
2. **Lower limbs.** Look at the skin on the patient's legs for leg ulcers, skin infections (e.g. boils) or pigmented scars. **Necrobiosis lipoidica diabeticorum** is a rare scarred lesion with a red margin and yellow centre that is usually found on the shins. Note any insulin injection site changes (causing fat atrophy or hypertrophy). Note any oedema.

   Examine for **neurological disease in the legs** (e.g. peripheral neuropathy, loss of proximal muscle power).

   Examine the peripheral pulses for loss. Feel the temperature of the feet and press the large toenail beds to test capillary return (**peripheral vascular disease**).
3. **The face.** Examine the patient's eyes. The fundi in particular need careful assessment for diabetic retinopathy (p. 145). Other signs can include a diabetic third cranial nerve palsy (typically with pupil sparing).
4. **The ears, nose and throat.** Look for any evidence of infection (e.g. fungal). Examine for a carotid bruit (carotid stenosis).
5. **The chest and abdomen.** Look for signs of infection. Palpate for hepatomegaly (fatty liver).
6. **Urinalysis.** Test for glucose and protein.
7. **Blood pressure.** Measure for postural hypotension (autonomic neuropathy).

The endocrine system: a systematic approach

Endocrine diseases can affect multiple organ systems. Some of the signs linked to the more important endocrine diseases are summarised here.

1. Pick up the patient's hands. Look at their overall size (increased in acromegaly—excess growth hormone) and for abnormalities of the nails (hyperthyroidism and hypothyroidism).
2. Take the patient's pulse (thyroid disease) and blood pressure (hypertension in Cushing's syndrome (glucocorticoid excess) or postural hypotension in Addison's disease (adrenocortical hypofunction)).
3. Look for Trousseau's sign (tetany from hypocalcaemia in hypoparathyroidism). Inflate the blood pressure cuff above systolic and wait 2 minutes: if positive, the thumb becomes adducted and the fingers extended.
4. Go to the axillae. Look for loss of axillary hair (pituitary failure: pan-hypopituitarism) or acanthosis nigricans and skin tags (acromegaly).
5. Examine the patient's eyes (hyperthyroidism) and the fundi (diabetes mellitus). Look at the face for hirsutism or fine-wrinkled hairless skin (pan-hypopituitarism). Note any skin greasiness, acne or plethora (Cushing's syndrome).
6. Look at the mouth for protrusion of the chin and enlargement of the tongue (acromegaly) or buccal pigmentation (Addison's disease).
7. Examine the neck for thyroid enlargement. Palpate for supraclavicular fat pads (Cushing's syndrome).
8. Inspect the chest wall for hirsutism or loss of body hair, reduction in breast size in women (pan-hypopituitarism). Look for gynaecomastia in men (e.g. testicular failure, thyrotoxicosis). Look for nipple pigmentation (Addison's disease).
9. Examine the abdomen for hirsutism, central fat deposition and purple striae (Cushing's syndrome). Look at the legs for diabetic changes.
10. Test the urine (diabetes mellitus).

The endocrine OSCE: hints panel

1 This woman has had thyrotoxicosis. Take a history from her.
  (a) Ask her the following:
   (i) How long is it since you became unwell?
   (ii) Do you feel back to normal now? How has the illness affected your life and work?
   (iii) Have you lost weight during this illness? How much?
   (iv) Have you found hot weather more uncomfortable than usual? Have you felt more anxious than before?
   (v) Have you had problems with diarrhoea?
   (vi) Have you had palpitations of the heart? What were they like?
   (vii) Have you had a goitre?
   (viii) Have you had problems with your eyes? What has happened to them? Has it improved?
   (ix) Is there thyroid trouble in your family?
   (x) What treatments have you had? Have any medications had to be stopped because of any problems?
  (b) Synthesise and present your findings.

2 This man has been diagnosed with hypothyroidism. Take a history from him.

(a) Ask him the following:
   (i)   How long have you been unwell?
   (ii) Do you feel back to normal now? How has the illness affected your life and work?
   (iii) Have you put on weight? How much?
   (iv) Have you found cold weather more intolerable than usual?
   (v)   Have you had problems with constipation?
   (vi) Have you had a goitre?
   (vii) Is there thyroid trouble in your family?
   (viii)What treatments have you had? Did any previous medications have to be stopped because of any problems?

(b) Synthesise and present your findings.

3 Please examine the eyes of this woman with thyrotoxicosis.

(a) Stand back to look for general abnormalities (tremor, apparent loss of weight, thyroid stare and the presence of a goitre).
(b) Look at the patient's eyes from in front and from above (looking over the forehead) for proptosis.
(c) Look at the conjunctivae for chemosis.
(d) Test for lid lag.
(e) Look for chemosis, conjunctivitis, corneal ulceration.
(f) Examine the fundi for optic atrophy if exophthalmos is present.
(g) Examine her eye movements in full (p. 119).
(h) Synthesise and present your findings.

4 Please take an appropriate history from this man who has had type 2 diabetes mellitus for 20 years.

(a) Ask him the following:
   (i)   How was your diabetes first diagnosed?
   (ii) What has happened to your weight since then?
   (iii) What type of diet are you on? Do you understand the reason for this type of diet?
   (iv) What medicines do you take for diabetes?
   (v)   Are you using insulin?
   (vi) Have you had hypoglycaemic episodes?
   (vii) How often do you test your blood sugar? Do you keep a record of your results? Has your sugar control been good?
   (viii)Have you had any problems with your vision? Do you have your eyes checked regularly? What have you been told about any complications involving your eyes?
   (ix) Have you had any kidney problems?
   (x)   Have you been told that you might have vascular problems involving the heart or be at risk of stroke?
   (xi) Do you smoke? Do you know what your cholesterol level is?
   (xii) Have you had any problems with dizziness on standing?
   (xiii)Have you had any problems with your digestion?
   (xiv)Have you had numbness in your fingers or toes?

(b) Synthesise and present your findings.

The endocrine system hints for success

1 Not all patients with thyroid disease will have a goitre. Careful examination of the neck for the presence of a goitre is part of the routine physical examination.

2 A thyroid that lies higher in the neck than average may appear enlarged but when it is not prominent enough to be palpable, there is unlikely to be a goitre.

3 Thyroid disease causes systemic symptoms and signs that are often of an insidious onset and may not be noticed by the patient or the patient's relatives.

4 Diabetics should be well informed about the complications of their disease. Every opportunity should be taken to remind them of the importance of careful blood sugar control and cardiovascular risk factor control.

5 Develop your own system for the complete examination of the diabetic patient.

6 Skin hyperpigmentation is a sign of Addison's disease (adrenocortical failure). Check for orthostatic hypotension.

chapter 10

The breasts

Breasts: Their use is to separate the milk for the nourishment of the foetus.
S Johnson, *A Dictionary Of The English Language* (1755)

Breast examination should be a routine part of the general physical examination.

The history

Ask whether the patient has presented for a routine breast examination or whether an abnormality has been noticed—many women regularly examine their own breasts for lumps. Other reasons for presenting include a bloody discharge from a nipple, breast pain or a request for assessment because of a family history of carcinoma of the breast in first- or second-degree relatives.

If the patient has noticed a lump, ask whether the lump is painful (rarely the case if the lump is malignant, but consider inflammatory carcinoma). Lumps that appear just before menstruation are likely to be hormonal and benign, but must be examined.

The occurrence of carcinoma in the other breast in the past is a strong risk factor for breast cancer. Breast carcinoma in two first-degree female relatives or one first-degree male relative, or bilateral breast cancer in one first-degree relative, are also important risk factors for breast cancer. Sometimes a relative will have been identified as having a specific gene associated with breast cancer.

Find out whether the patient has had a previous breast biopsy. The biopsied area may feel firm or lumpy. A previous biopsy may have shown atypical ductal hyperplasia, which is considered a premalignant condition.

Take a hormonal history, noting the age of menarche, the age of menopause (if relevant), the age of the first full-term pregnancy (if relevant) and whether the children were breastfed. Also ask about exogenous hormone use, including the contraceptive pill. All these factors may influence the risk of breast cancer.

Examination of the breasts
Inspection

Ask the patient to sit up with her chest fully exposed. Look at the nipples for retraction (due to **cancer** or fibrosis; note in some patients retraction may be normal) and **Paget's disease** of the nipple (where underlying breast cancer causes a unilateral red, scaling or bleeding area).

Inspect the rest of the skin. Look for **visible veins** (which, if unilateral, suggest a cancer), skin **dimpling** and peau d'orange skin (where advanced breast cancer causes oedematous skin pitted by the sweat glands).

Ask the patient to **raise her arms above her head**. Look for tethering of the nipples or skin, a shift in the relative position of the nipples or a fixed mass distorting the breast. Look for axillary lumps.

Ask the patient to rest her hands on her hips and then press her hands against her hips (the **pectoral contraction manoeuvre**). This accentuates areas of dimpling or fixation.

Palpation

Make sure your hands are clean and warm. Ask the patient to lie down. It can be helpful to have her place her hand, for the same side, behind her head.

Feel each breast systematically (see Fig 10.1). Palpation is performed gently with the pulps of the middle three fingers parallel to the contour of the breast. The total examination should involve a rectangular area bordered by the clavicle, the sternum, the mid-axillary line and the bra line. Start in the axilla and palpate in a line down to the bra line inferiorly. The pattern of palpation is like that of mowing a lawn, a series of vertical strips that cover the whole of the rectangle. Each area is palpated three times, using small circular movements and slightly increasing pressure.

Next, feel **behind the nipple** for lumps and note whether any **fluid** can be expressed: bright blood (e.g. from a duct papilloma or, more rarely, a carcinoma), yellow serous fluid (e.g. fibroadenosis) or serous fluid (e.g. early pregnancy), milky fluid (e.g. lactation) or green fluid (e.g. mammary duct ectasia).

The presence of breast implants makes the examination much more difficult. The patient's ipsilateral arm should then be kept down at her side and the breast examined while she lies supine.

Examine both the **supraclavicular** and **axillary** regions for lymphadenopathy (p. 102).

Evaluation of a breast lump

The following points need to be carefully elucidated if a lump is detected.
- *Position:* the breast quadrant involved and proximity to the nipple.
- *Size, shape and consistency:* a hard, irregular nodule is characteristic of carcinoma.
- *Tenderness:* suggests an inflammatory or cystic lesion; breast cancer is usually not tender.

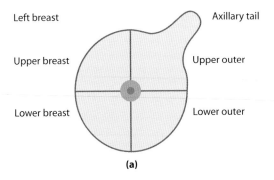

Left breast

Axillary tail

Upper breast

Upper outer

Lower breast

Lower outer

(a)

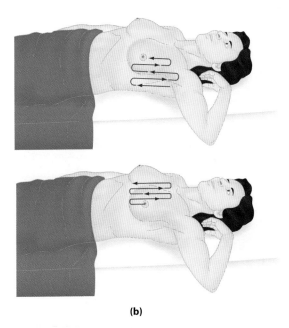

(b)

Figure 10.1 Examination of the breast: **(a)** quadrants; **(b)** systematic examination

- *Fixation:* mobility is determined by taking the breast between the hands and moving it over the chest wall with the arm relaxed and then with the hand pressing on the hip (to tense the pectoralis major). For lower outer quadrant lesions the arm should push against a wall in front of the patient (to tense the serratus anterior muscle). In advanced carcinoma the lump may be fixed to the chest wall.
- *Single or multiple lesions:* multiple nodules suggest benign cystic disease or fibroadenosis.

- *Lymph node enlargement:* examine the **draining** axillary and supraclavicular lymph nodes—the presence of nodes suggests metastatic disease.

If carcinoma is suspected, examine for metastatic disease (see the box on p. 99). Examine for a pleural effusion. Check for vertebral or other bony tenderness. Palpate for a hard, irregular liver (malignant hepatomegaly).

The male breasts

In men with true gynaecomastia (breast tissue enlargement), a disc of breast tissue can be palpated under the areola. This is not present in men who are merely obese.

Breast examination hints for success

1 Examination of the female breasts is a routine aspect of physical examination.
2 The examination is not complete unless the draining lymph nodes are also examined.
3 Examine for evidence of distant metastases if carcinoma is suspected.

chapter 11

The joints

Rheumatism: A painful distemper supposed to proceed from acrid humours.

S Johnson, *A Dictionary Of The English Language* (1755)

Joint abnormalities are commonly due to injury, inflammation or degeneration (wear and tear). Inflammatory joint conditions are often associated with abnormalities of the skin and connective tissues.

The rheumatological history

Presenting symptoms (see Table 11.1)

Table 11.1 Rheumatological history: presenting symptoms
Major symptoms
Joints   Pain   Swelling   Morning stiffness   Loss of function
Back pain
Limb pain
Eyes   Dry eyes and mouth   Red eyes
Raynaud's phenomenon
Systemic and other symptoms   Rash, fever, fatigue, weight loss, diarrhoea, mucosal ulcers

Joint pain and swelling

Ask the patient what joint problems have occurred. *Arthralgia* refers to joint pain without swelling, whereas *arthritis* means both pain and swelling. Determine whether one or many joints are involved, whether the symptoms are of an acute or chronic nature and whether they are getting better or worse. Patients with rheumatoid arthritis have **joint symptoms that are worse after rest**, whereas those with osteoarthritis have **pain that is worse after exercise**. Ask about **early morning stiffness**, which is a symptom of active synovitis (inflammation of the synovium).

Ask detailed questions about the ability of the patient with arthritis to perform usual activities at home and at work (p. 18).

Back pain

This is a very common complaint. Musculoskeletal pain is characteristically well localised and is aggravated by movement. If there is a spinal cord lesion there may be pain that occurs in a dermatomal distribution (see Fig 7.13). Diseases such as osteoporosis (with crush fractures), osteomalacia or infiltration of carcinoma, leukaemia or myeloma may cause progressive and unremitting back pain. The pain may be of sudden onset if it results from the crush fracture of a vertebral body. In **ankylosing spondylitis** (an inflammatory arthritis of the axial skeleton), the pain is usually situated over the sacroiliac joints and lumbar spine and is improved by exercise; early morning stiffness accompanies the pain.

Limb pain

This can occur from disease of the musculoskeletal system (including trauma), skin, vascular system or nervous system. Pain and stiffness in the shoulders and hips in patients over the age of 50 years may be due to **polymyalgia rheumatica**. Bone disease, such as osteomyelitis, osteomalacia, osteoporosis or tumours, can cause limb pain. Inflammation of tendons (tenosynovitis) can produce local pain over the affected area.

Vascular disease may also produce pain in the limbs. Consider arterial occlusion if there has been severe pain of sudden onset. Chronic peripheral vascular disease can result in calf pain on exercise that is relieved by rest. This is called *intermittent claudication*. Venous thrombosis can also cause diffuse aching pain in the legs associated with swelling.

Associated symptoms

Dry eyes and mouth

Dry eyes and dry mouth are characteristic of Sjögren's syndrome, which is an autoimmune disease. The dry eyes can result in conjunctivitis, keratitis and corneal ulcers.

Red eyes

The seronegative (rheumatoid factor is not present in the blood) spondyloarthropathies and Behçet's syndrome, but not rheumatoid arthritis, may be complicated by iritis (as described on p. 146).

Raynaud's phenomenon

Raynaud's phenomenon is an abnormal vascular response of the exposed fingers (and toes) to cold; the fingers first turn white, then blue and finally become red and painful.

Systemic and other symptoms

Ask about rashes and mucosal ulcers. In patients with back pain, serious spinal pathology should be suspected if there are 'red flag' features (e.g. fever, neurological symptoms or faecal incontinence, weight loss).

Past history

It is important to ask about any history of trauma or surgery. Similarly, a history of recent infection, including hepatitis, streptococcal pharyngitis, rubella, dysentery, gonorrhoea and tuberculosis, may be relevant in determining the cause of arthralgia or arthritis. Inflammatory bowel disease causing bloody diarrhoea can also result in arthritis.

Social history

Determine the patient's domestic set-up and occupation. This is particularly relevant if a chronic, disabling arthritis has developed.

Treatment history

Document current and previous anti-arthritic medications (e.g. aspirin, COX-2 selective inhibitors, other NSAIDs, gold, methotrexate, salazopyrin, chloroquine, steroids, anti-tumour necrosis factor (TNF) drugs). Any side effects of these drugs also need to be ascertained. Enquire about physiotherapy and joint surgery in the past.

Family history

Some diseases associated with chronic arthritis run in families. For example, rheumatoid arthritis is four times more common in people who have an affected first-degree relative.

The rheumatological examination
General inspection

A general inspection gives an indication of the patient's functional disability and allows the 'spot diagnosis' of certain conditions. Look at the patient walking into the room and note apparent pain and difficulty, the posture and whether there is the need for mechanical assistance. Observe the pattern of joint involvement (which joints, and whether symmetrical or not).

Position the patient for a more detailed examination, in bed and undressed as far as practical. Watch for any difficulty the patient may have in undressing.

The principles of joint examination

Look, **feel**, **move** and **measure** when examining the affected joints.

1. Look (compare right with left) for:
   - **Erythema:** redness of overlying skin suggests active **arthritis** or **infection** of the joint.
   - **Atrophy:** wasting of skin and its appendages suggests the condition is chronic.
   - **Scars:** previous operations may have been performed on the joint or associated tendons (e.g. joint replacement or tendon repair).
   - **Rashes:** (1) psoriasis, a scaly, silvery rash on the extensor tendons, is associated with a number of types of arthritis; (2) vasculitis, which is inflammation of small arteries, causes skin (e.g. palpable purpura) and nail bed changes (e.g. linear haemorrhages) and can be associated with active arthritis (e.g. rheumatoid arthritis).
   - **Swelling** over the joint: this may be due to effusion (fluid accumulation within the joint space), hypertrophy or inflammation of the synovium (boggy swelling), or to bony overgrowths at the joint margins (hard swelling in osteoarthritis).
   - **Deformity:** destructive arthritis causes distortion of the architecture of the area involved (e.g. the deviation of the fingers towards the ulnar side of the hand in severe rheumatoid arthritis).
   - **Subluxation:** displaced parts of the joint surfaces remain partly in contact.
   - **Dislocation:** loss of contact between the joint surfaces occurs as a result of damage to the joint surfaces and the surrounding tissues and tendons.
   - **Muscle wasting:** disuse, inflammation and sometimes nerve entrapment can all be responsible for the wasting of muscles near affected joints.

2. Feel for:
   - **Warmth:** active synovitis, infection or crystal arthritis (e.g. gout) all cause increased vascularity and make the area around the affected joint warmer than normal.
   - **Tenderness:** joint inflammation or infection is a likely cause.
   - **Synovitis:** this causes a very characteristic boggy swelling that is firmer than an effusion.
   - **Bony swelling:** osteophyte formation or subchondral bone thickening is very hard.

3. Move:
   - **Passive** movement: ask the patient to relax and let you move the joint in its normal anatomical directions; note limited extension (called **fixed flexion deformity**) or limited flexion (called **fixed extension deformity**).
   - **Active** movement: to assess integrated joint function (e.g. hand function, gait, neck and back examination), ask the patient to move the joint.

- **Stability:** attempt to move the joint gently in abnormal directions; an unstable joint can be moved in directions other than its usual planes of movement because of dislocation or loss of normal tendon support.
- **Joint crepitus:** place your hand over the joint or tendons as the patient moves the joint—a grating sensation or noise from the joint suggests chronicity.

4. Measure:
   - **Estimate** the approximate joint angles. Record movement as the number of degrees of flexion from the anatomical position in extension (e.g. straight knee). A knee with a fixed flexion deformity may be recorded as 30° to 60°, which indicates that there is 30° of fixed flexion deformity and that flexion is limited to 60°.
   - **Use a tape measure** (1) to measure and follow serially the quadriceps muscle bulk and (2) in examination of spinal movements (see below).

Examination of individual joints

You must know how to fully examine the hands, back and knees, although other joints also can provide important diagnostic information.

The hands and wrists

Examination anatomy

The complex functions of the hand are reflected in the complexity of the wrist and hand joints (see Fig 11.1). The wrist comprises two synovial joints: the radiocarpal joint (between the radial head and the proximal carpal bones) and the midcarpal joint (between the two rows of carpal bones). Lateral and medial collateral ligaments and anterior and posterior ligaments stabilise the joint surfaces during different movements. Wrist movements include ulnar and lateral deviation and flexion and extension. A combination of these movements results in circumduction of the hand.

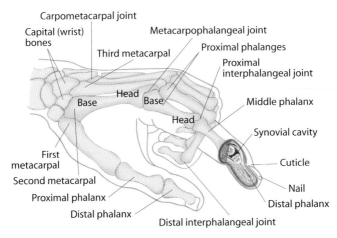

Figure 11.1 Anatomy of the hand and wrist

The carpometacarpal joints connect the wrist and the hand. These are condyloid synovial joints. Movement can occur around two axes at right angles to each other: flexion and extension, and adduction and abduction. The carpometacarpal joint of the thumb (between the first metacarpal bone and the trapezium) has more complicated articular surfaces. These allow a greater range of movements: flexion, extension, adduction, abduction, rotation and circumduction.

The metacarpophalangeal joints are synovial joints. Possible active movements include flexion, extension, abduction, adduction and some rotation. Extension is much more limited than flexion. The movement of the metacarpophalangeal joint of the thumb is again different. This joint is mostly limited to flexion and extension.

Examination of the hands and wrists
Sit the patient over the side of the bed and place the patient's hands on the pillow with the palms down.

1. Look:
   - **Wrists:** note erythema, atrophy, scars, swelling and rashes; also look for hollow ridges between the metacarpal bones (muscle wasting of the intrinsic muscles of the hand).
   - **Metacarpophalangeal joints:** note skin abnormalities, swelling or deformity (ulnar deviation and volar (palmar) subluxation of the fingers).
   - **Proximal interphalangeal** and **distal interphalangeal joints:** note skin changes and joint swelling.
   - **Swan neck deformity**; note flexion of proximal interphalangeal joints and hyperextension of distal interphalangeal joints: this is characteristic of rheumatoid arthritis (see Fig 11.2(b)).
   - **Osteoarthritis:** note the presence of **swollen** distal interphalangeal and first carpometacarpal joints. Look for **Heberden's nodes**, which are marginal osteophytes that lie at the base of the distal phalanx.
   - **Fingers:** note the presence of the **typical sausage-shaped fingers** of psoriatic arthropathy.
   - **Nails:** note **psoriatic** nail changes such as pitting (see Fig 3.3), onycholysis, hyperkeratosis (thickened nails), ridging and discolouration.
   - **Vasculitic** changes: look for linear haemorrhages (e.g. due to rheumatoid arthritis).
   - **Palmar surfaces**: note scars (from tendon repairs or transfers), palmar erythema and muscle wasting of the thenar or hypothenar eminences.
2. Feel and move (see Fig 11.2(a)):
   - Feel with your two thumbs at the **wrists** for **synovitis** (see Fig 11.2(c)) and effusions. Note tenderness, limitation of movement or joint crepitus.
   - Go on to the metacarpophalangeal joints. **Flex the metacarpophalangeal joint** with the proximal phalanx held between the thumb and forefinger, then rock the joint backwards and forwards.

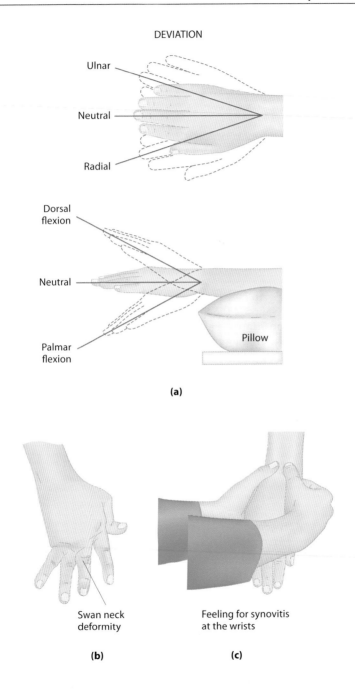

Figure 11.2 (a) Movements of the hands and wrists **(b)** Swan neck deformity **(c)** Feeling for synovitis at the wrists

Considerable movement may be present when ligamentous laxity or subluxation is present.

- **Palpate all the proximal and distal interphalangeal joints** for tenderness and swelling. Bony swelling is hard and due to the presence of osteophytes.
- Test for **palmar tendon crepitus**. Place the palmar aspects of your fingers against the palm of the patient's hand while he or she flexes and extends the metacarpophalangeal joints. Look for a **trigger finger** (inability to extend a finger in stenosing tenosynovitis).
- Perform **Finkelstein's test**. Hold the patient's hand with the thumb tucked into the palm and then turn the wrist quickly into full ulnar deviation. Sharp pain will occur in the thumb tendons when there is tenosynovitis of these tendons (de Quervain's tenosynovitis).
- Feel for the **subcutaneous nodules** of rheumatoid arthritis near the elbows.

3. Test for function:
   - Test for **grip strength** by getting the patient to squeeze two of your fingers.
   - Test for **key grip** (see Fig 11.3) by getting the patient to hold a key between the pulps of the thumb and forefinger.
   - Test for **opposition strength** (see Fig 11.3) by asking the patient to oppose the thumb and little finger, then assess the difficulty with which these can be forced apart.
   - Perform a **practical test**, such as asking the patient to undo a button or write with a pen.

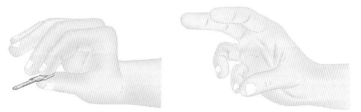

Figure 11.3 The key grip and testing opposition strength

The elbows

1. Look for a **joint effusion** (a swelling on either side of the olecranon). Discrete swellings over the olecranon may be due to rheumatoid nodules (firm swellings that may be tender and are attached to deeper structures), gouty tophi or an enlarged olecranon bursa.
2. Feel for **tenderness**, particularly over the epicondyles. **Rheumatoid nodules** are hard, may be tender and are attached to underlying structures, whereas **gouty tophi** have a firm feeling and often appear yellow-coloured under the skin.
3. Move the elbow joints passively. The elbow is a hinge joint with movement from 0° (**extension**) to 150° (**flexion**) (see Fig 11.4).

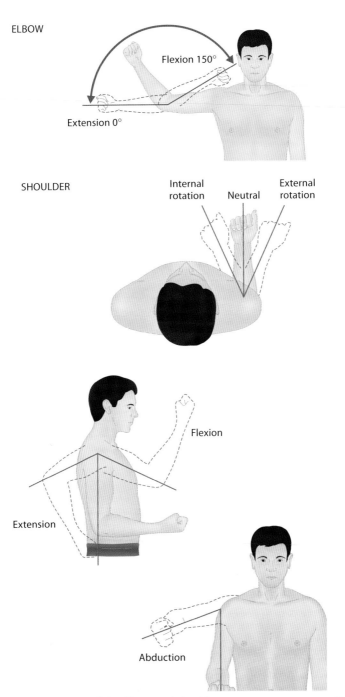

ELBOW

Flexion 150°

Extension 0°

SHOULDER

Internal rotation   Neutral   External rotation

Flexion

Extension

Abduction

Figure 11.4 Movements of the elbows and shoulders   *continued*

SHOULDER

In abduction:

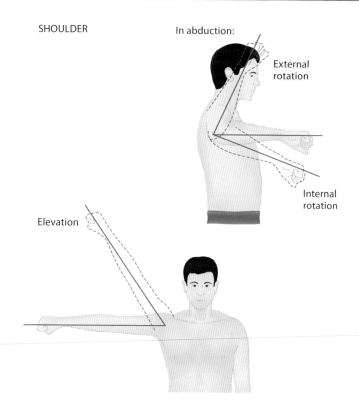

Figure 11.4 Movements of the elbows and shoulders *continued*

The shoulders

1. Look at the joint. Only large effusions can be detected.
2. Feel for tenderness and swelling.
3. Move the joint passively. Test **abduction** (90°), **elevation** (180°), **adduction** (50°), **external rotation** (60°), **internal rotation** (90°), **flexion** (180°) and **extension** (65°) (see Fig 11.4).

The temporomandibular joints

1. Look in front of the ear for swelling.
2. Feel for grating and tenderness, by placing a finger just in front of the ear while the patient opens and shuts the mouth.

The neck

1. Look at the cervical spine while the patient is sitting up and note particularly the patient's posture.
2. Test **movement** actively for **flexion** (45°), **extension** (45°), **lateral bending** (45°) and **rotation** (70°) (see Fig 11.5).

NECK

Rotation

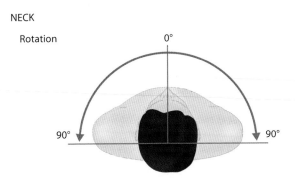

Anteroposterior

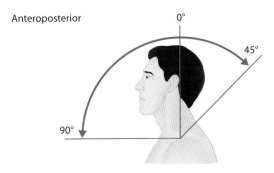

Lateral

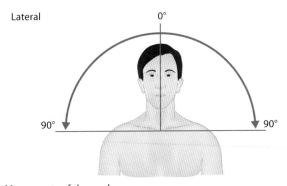

Figure 11.5 Movements of the neck

The thoracolumbar spine and sacroiliac joints

To start the examination, have the patient standing and clothed only in underwear.

1. Look for **deformity** such as scoliosis, a lateral curvature of the spine or loss of the normal thoracic kyphosis (see Fig 11.6), and lumbar lordosis (e.g. due to ankylosing spondylitis).

2. Feel **each vertebral body** for tenderness and palpate for muscle spasm. Also feel for sacroiliac joint tenderness (see Fig 11.6).

3. Test movement actively: **flexion, extension, lateral bending** and **rotation** (see Fig 11.6).

Assess **straight leg raising**, with the patient lying down, by lifting the straightened leg. In lumbar disc prolapse (L4, L5, S1 nerve roots) this will be limited by pain.

Perform the **femoral nerve stretch test**. Ask the patient to lie on his or her front (prone). Flex the knee then extend the hip. Pain in the back (or front of the thigh) is a positive test (p. 142).

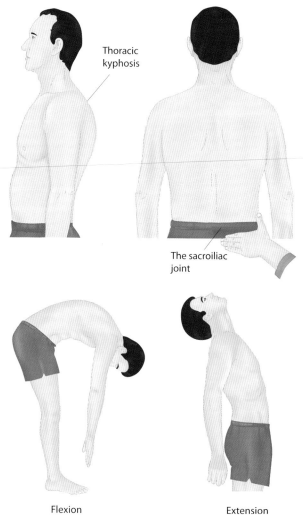

Thoracic kyphosis

The sacroiliac joint

Flexion

Extension

Figure 11.6 Movements of the thoracolumbar spine

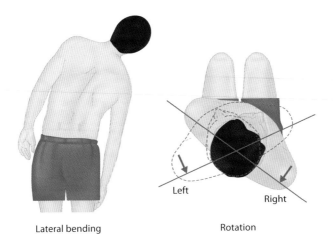

Lateral bending   Rotation

Figure 11.6 Movements of the thoracolumbar spine con*tinued*

The hips

1. Feel just distal to the midpoint of the inguinal ligament for joint tenderness.
2. Move the hip joint passively with the patient lying down, first on the back.
3. Test **flexion** (90°), **abduction** (50°) and **adduction** (45°). Ask the patient to roll over onto the stomach and test **extension**, **external rotation** and **internal rotation** (45°) (see Fig 11.7).

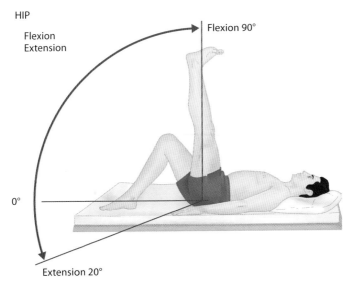

Figure 11.7 Movements of the hip   *continued*

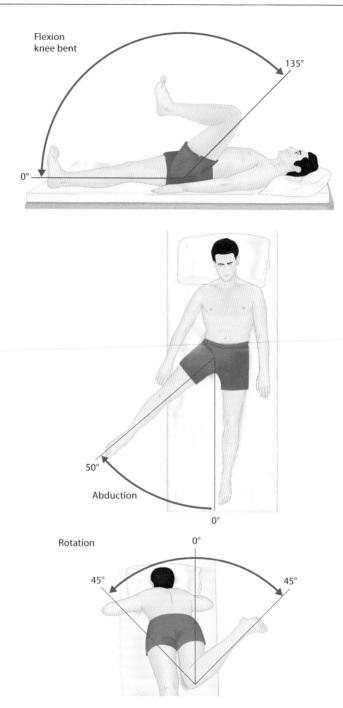

Figure 11.7 Movements of the hip *continued*

4. Ask the patient to stand and perform the **Trendelenburg test**. The patient stands first on one leg and then on the other. Normally the non-weightbearing hip rises, but with proximal myopathy or hip joint disease the non-weightbearing side sags.

The knees

Examination anatomy

The knee is the largest hinge joint in the body (see Fig 11.8). It has a large synovium and collateral ligaments to provide lateral stability and cruciate ligaments to limit movement in the antero-posterior direction. Examination of the knee must assess these complex structures.

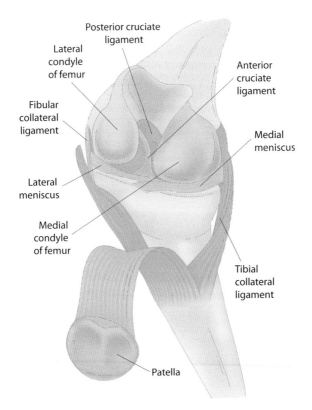

Figure 11.8 Anatomy of the knee

Examination of the knees

1. Look for quadriceps wasting and examine the knees themselves for skin changes, swelling and deformity. A space will be visible under the knee if there is a permanent flexion deformity.
2. Feel the quadriceps for **wasting**. Palpate over the knees for warmth and synovial swelling.

3. Use the **patellar tap** to confirm the presence of large effusions. Compress the lower end of the quadriceps muscle and push any fluid contained in the suprapatellar bursa down and under the patella. Use your other hand to push down briskly on the patella. The presence of posterior displacement of the patella followed by a tap is a sign of a significant fluid collection.

4. Move the joint passively. Test **flexion** (135°) and **extension** (5°), and note the presence of crepitus (see Fig 11.9(a)).

5. Test the **collateral** and **cruciate ligaments** (see Fig 11.9 (b) and (c)). The lateral and medial collateral ligaments are tested by having the patient flex the knee slightly. Rest your arm along the patient's tibia and attempt lateral and medial movements of the leg on the knee. The thigh is steadied with your other hand. Movement of more than 10° is abnormal. The cruciate ligaments are tested by flexing the patient's knee to 90°. One hand steadies the thigh while the other, placed behind the patient's knee, attempts to produce anterior and posterior movements of the leg on the knee joint.

6. Finally, stand the patient up. Look particularly for **varus** (bow leg) and **valgus** (knock-knee) deformity. Look and feel behind the knees in the **popliteal fossa** for a Baker's cyst.

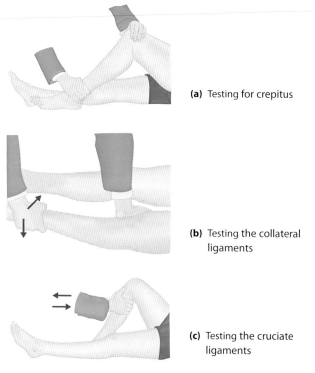

(a) Testing for crepitus

(b) Testing the collateral ligaments

(c) Testing the cruciate ligaments

Figure 11.9 Examining the knee joints

The ankles and feet

1. Look at the skin for swelling, deformity (hallux valgus and clawing) or muscle wasting. **Sausage-like deformities of the toes** occur with psoriatic arthropathy, ankylosing spondylitis and Reiter's disease. Look for the nail changes that suggest psoriasis. Inspect the transverse arch of the foot and the longitudinal arch; these may be flattened in arthritic conditions of the foot.
2. Feel for **swelling** around the lateral and medial malleoli.
3. Move the **talar (ankle) joint**, grasping the mid-foot with one hand (**dorsiflexion** and **plantar flexion**).
4. With the **subtalar joint**, tenderness on movement is more important than range of movement.
5. Squeeze the **metatarsophalangeal joints** by compressing the first and fifth metatarsals between your thumb and forefinger. Tenderness suggests inflammation.
6. Palpate the **Achilles tendon** for rheumatoid nodules or Achilles tendonitis.

The joints OSCE: hints panel

1 **This woman has rheumatoid arthritis. Please take a history from her to assess the severity of the disease and its affect on her.**
   (a) Ask her the following:
      (i)   How old are you? How old were you at the onset of the disease?
      (ii)   What joints have been involved and at roughly what times?
      (iii) Do you currently have any active arthritis (morning stiffness, swelling)? What joints?
      (iv)   What has been and is your occupation? How do you cope at work? Do you feel confident about continuing to work?
      (v)   Can you drive? How do you manage bathing, dressing, toileting, etc?
      (vi)   Who lives at home with you? How do these people cope with your illness?
      (vii) Has your house or car had to be modified? Do you need a walking stick, frame or wheelchair?
      (viii) What treatment are you on? Have you required steroids? What problems have the drugs caused? Have you required treatment for osteoporosis or anaemia?
      (ix)   Have you had joint or tendon surgery?
      (x)   Are you concerned about your future health?
   (b) Synthesise and present your findings.

2 **This patient has painful hands. Please examine them.**
   (a) Stand back to look at the patient for obvious generalised arthritis.
   (b) Get him to sit up in a chair or with his legs over the edge of the bed and rest his hands on a pillow.
   (c) Look at the palmar and dorsal surfaces before touching his hands. Note the various deformities described on p. 173.
   (d) Ask whether there are any areas of tenderness.
   (e) Examine his hands as outlined on p. 172.
   (f) Present your findings at the end, or describe any abnormalities as you go along.

3   This patient has right knee pain on walking. Please examine him.
   (a) Ask the patient to expose *both* his legs to at least the mid-thigh.
   (b) Test gait. Look from the front and sides.
   (c) While the patient gets back on the bed stand back and look for more general abnormalities including deformities of other major joints.
   (d) Now inspect his knees. Look for obvious signs of inflammation or deformity. Is there an obvious effusion?
   (e) Ask whether his knees are tender. Feel his knees. Note any tenderness and the skin temperature.
   (f) Assess knee movements, crepitus and ligament stability.
   (g) Synthesise and present your findings.

4   This man has had lower back pain. Please examine his back.
   (a) Ask the patient to undress to his underpants.
   (b) Watch him undressing for problems with immobility or pain.
   (c) Look at his back for deformity (increased or reduced thoracic kyphosis or lumbar lordosis, scoliosis) and for scars from previous back surgery.
   (d) Ask about tenderness. Palpate each vertebral body and the sacroiliac joints. Use your closed fist to gently percuss for tenderness.
   (e) Test the range of movements, asking whether movement is painful each time ('touch your toes with straight legs', 'lean back as far as possible', 'reach down to the side and touch below your knee').
   (f) Ask the patient to lie in bed and perform straight leg raising and the femoral nerve stretch test.
   (g) Synthesise and present your findings.

5   Please assess this woman's hand function.
   (a) Look at her hands for deformity and swelling.
   (b) Ask whether they are tender.
   (c) Ask her to perform various tasks to test hand function: key grip (opposition and adduction of thumb), pinch grip (opposition and flexion of thumb) and dressing (hand, elbow, shoulder).
   (d) Ask to perform a neurological examination of the hand for peripheral nerve or sensory lesions.
   (e) Synthesise and present your findings.

Examination of the joints   hints for success

1   Ask about pain and stiffness in all the joints.
2   Determine the actual joint involvement by history and confirm this on examination.
3   Always compare an affected joint with the opposite joint to ascertain the amount of abnormality.
4   Inflamed joints are usually hot, red, swollen and tender. Impaired function is also present.
5   Functional assessment of involved joints gives important information about the clinical impact of a condition.
6   Distinguishing non-specific lower back pain from that of ankylosing spondylitis is difficult, but tenderness to pressure over the sacroiliac joints is a helpful sign of the latter.

chapter 12

The skin

Specialist—A man who knows more and more about less and less.
William James Mayo (1861–1934)

The dermatological history

The patient may have presented because of concern about a skin problem, or a lesion or an abnormality may have been noticed during examination. In either case, certain questions should be asked:

1. How long has the lesion or abnormality been present?
2. Has its distribution changed over time?
3. Has it been associated with sun exposure or exposure to heat or cold?
4. Is there associated pruritus (itch)? Itch can be due to local skin disease (e.g. dry skin, atopic dermatitis, scabies) or a systemic disease (e.g. obstructive jaundice, chronic renal failure, lymphoma).
5. Is the lesion painful or associated with altered sensation?
6. Does the patient have constitutional symptoms (fever, loss of weight, headache etc)?
7. Does the patient have a past history of skin disease or atopy (allergy)?
8. Does the patient have a history of systemic disease (e.g. inflammatory bowel disease, diabetes mellitus, connective tissue disease, arthritis)?
9. Does the patient have a history of exposure to chemicals, animals or plants?
10. Does the patient have a family history of melanoma? (10% of melanomas)
11. What medications is the patient taking?

Examination anatomy

Figure 12.1 shows the three main layers of the skin: the epidermis, dermis and subcutaneous fat. These layers can all be involved in skin diseases in varying combinations. Most skin tumours arise in the epidermis. Skin appendages such as hair follicles (see Fig 12.2) are a common site of infection, especially in adolescents and people on steroid medications (acne).

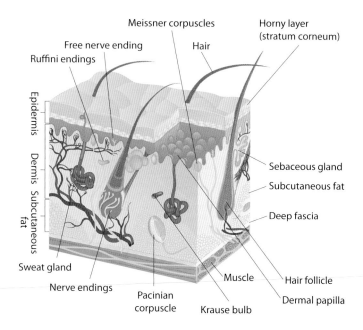

Figure 12.1 The three main layers of the skin

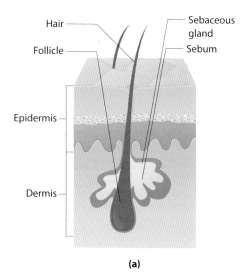

(a)

Figure 12.2 (a) Clear skin

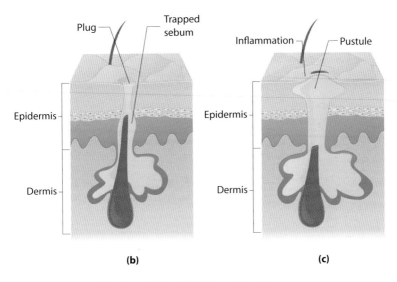

Figure 12.2 (b) Blackhead **(c)** Infected follicle *continued*

Examination of the skin

The patient should undress so that the whole surface of the skin is accessible. First, any lesions must be **described** precisely according to their colour and shape and using dermatological terms (see Table 12.1). Then their **distribution** must be noted and the **pattern** of the lesions must be described (see Table 12.2). Finally, the lesions should be **palpated** (p. 32), noting consistency, tenderness, temperature, depth within the skin and mobility of any lesion and the skin overlying it.

Table 12.1 **Dermatological terms**	
Atrophy	thinning of epidermis with loss of normal skin markings
Bulla	a larger collection of fluid below the epidermis
Crust	dried serum and exudate
Ecchymoses	bruises
Excoriations	lesions caused by scratching that results in loss of the epidermis
Keloid	hypertrophic scaring
Macule	a circumscribed alteration of skin colour
Nodule	a circumscribed palpable mass greater than 1 cm in diameter

continued

Table 12.1 Dermatological terms *continued*

Papule	a circumscribed palpable elevation less than 1 cm in diameter
Petechiae	red non-blanching spots < 5 mm
Pigment alterations	increased (hyperpigmentation) or decreased (hypopigmentation)
Plaque	a palpable disc-shaped lesion
Purpura	red non-blanching spots > 5 mm
Pustule	a visible collection of pus
Scales	an accumulation of excess keratin
Sclerosis	induration of subcutaneous tissues that may involve the dermis
Ulcer	a circumscribed loss of tissue
Vesicle	a small collection of fluid below the epidermis
Wheal	an area of dermal oedema

Table 12.2 Patterns in dermatology

Annular	ring-shaped (hollow centre), e.g. tinea infection
Arcuate	curved, e.g. secondary syphilis
Circinate	circular
Confluent	lesions that have run together, e.g. measles
Discoid	circular without a hollow centre, e.g. lupus
Eczematous	inflamed and crusted, e.g. allergic eczema
Keratotic	thickened from increased keratin, e.g. psoriasis
Lichenified	thickening and roughening of the epidermis associated with accentuated skin markings
Linear	in lines, e.g. contact dermatitis
Nodule	raised solid lesion > 10 mm, e.g. erythema nodosum
Papule	raised solid lesion < 10 mm, e.g. wart
Papulosquamous	plaques associated with scaling
Reticulated	in a network pattern, e.g. cutaneous parasite
Serpiginous	sinuous
Zosteriform	following a nerve distribution

Skin tumours

Skin tumours are very common skin lesions. Most are benign, but malignant tumours must be recognised early (see box below), because successful treatment depends on early diagnosis.

Skin tumours

1 Solar keratoses (actinic)—premalignant
2 Basal cell carcinoma
3 Squamous cell carcinoma
4 Bowen's disease (squamous cell carcinoma confined to the epithelial layer of the skin—carcinoma in situ)
5 Malignant melanoma
6 Secondary deposits

Primary skin cancers of all types are more common in people with fair skin who have been exposed to the sun. Many cancers will eventually ulcerate. All non-healing ulcers should be considered malignant until proved benign.

Solar keratoses are premalignant. They may begin as pink macules often surrounded by adherent scale. They often feel rough, like sand paper. A proportion of them regress spontaneously. **Basal cell carcinomas** begin as a papule with a depressed centre and have a rolled border that has a characteristic pearly appearance (see Fig 12.3(a)). **Squamous cell carcinomas** begin as an opaque papule or plaque that is often eroded or scaly. **Malignant melanomas** often appear as deeply pigmented lesions with an irregular border (see Fig 12.3(b)). They enlarge and often develop patchy changes in pigment colour.

Figure 12.3 (a) Basal cell carcinoma   *continued*

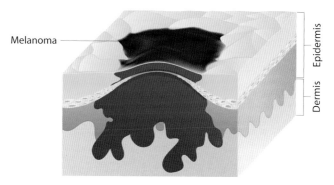

Figure 12.3 (b) Melanoma *continued*

Remember to note the features on the ABCD checklist (see box below).

Melanomas (ABCD checklist)

- Are typically **A**symmetrical.
- Have an irregular **B**order.
- Have an irregular **C**olour.
- Can be large in **D**iameter.

The skin OSCE: hints panel

This man has a pigmented lesion on his chest. Please assess him.

(a) Ask him the following:
  (i)   Did you have any sun exposure in childhood? As an adult?
  (ii) Do you have a family history of melanoma?
  (iii) When did you first notice the lesion? Is it new?
  (iv) Has the lesion changed in appearance?
  (v)   Do you have any itching or bleeding?
  (vi) Have you had this lesion, or any other pigmented lesion, biopsied or excised?
(b) Inspect the lesion. Note whether it is symmetrical or not, has a regular or irregular border, is raised or not and has uniform or variable pigmentation, and look for any ulceration or inflammation. Measure the lesion's size.
(c) Inspect the skin all over his body, including in his hair, for other pigmented lesions.
(d) Note the features on the ABCD checklist (melanomas are typically asymmetrical, have an irregular border, have an irregular colour and can be large in diameter).
(e) If this could be a melanoma, request a surgical biopsy.
(f) Synthesise and present your findings.

chapter 13

Assessment of the geriatric patient

Age is an issue of mind over matter. If you don't mind, it doesn't matter.

Samuel Clemens (Mark Twain) (1835–1910)

Generally defined as individuals aged 65 years or older, geriatric patients tend to report fewer symptoms but have more numerous chronic diseases. Disease presentation is more likely to be atypical, so spending time taking the history is critical. Patients may have hearing loss, difficulty seeing and cognitive impairment, which can all impair history taking here.

History taking in the geriatric patient: special considerations

1. **Presenting symptoms:** these are usually multiple.
2. **Past history:** the immunisation status, especially for pneumococcus, influenza, tetanus and varicella zoster, should be recorded.
3. **Medications:** many patients will be taking multiple medications for several diseases, not all of which they may really need (polypharmacy). A comprehensive list, including reason for use, is important in terms of planning management.
4. **Social history:**
   - **Smoking habits:** details should be acquired as usual. Quitting smoking improves lung function, even in patients over the age of 60. Furthermore, advice to stop smoking is as successful in older patients as it is in younger ones.
   - **Exercise:** exercise is generally safe in the elderly and improves flexibility, balance, endurance and strength, which can assist with maintenance of independent function as well as improving quality of life.
   - **Living arrangements:** ask whether there is someone to help the patient in the home, if required.

- **Vulnerability:** abuse and neglect can be problems in this age group. Try to find out whether the patient feels under threat from anyone.
5. **Review of systems:**
   - Focus especially on vision, hearing, chewing and dentition, weight change, stool and urinary incontinence, recurrent falls, history of fractures and foot disease.
   - Find out whether the patient has had a problem with falls, and particularly if any injuries have occurred. Falls are an important cause of mortality in the elderly and are usually multi-factorial: postural dizziness, poor vision, cognitive impairment, foot problems, impaired bone mineral density and gait problems can all contribute to or exacerbate the problem. A history of falls means that careful enquiry must be made about these associated factors.
   - Ask about symptoms of depression, because this is a common problem in the elderly and needs to be recognised and treated.
6. **Specific areas of enquiry:**
   - **Physical activities of daily living (ADLs):** ask the patient how he or she copes with bathing, dressing, toileting and handling money—these can be affected by many different chronic illnesses.
   - **Instrumental activities of daily living (IADLs):** ask the patient whether he or she has any difficulty using the telephone, shopping, preparing food, housekeeping, doing the laundry, driving and taking medicines.
   - **End-of-life and treatment decisions:** patients generally prefer their clinician to actively bring up this topic. It is worth encouraging the patient to write down his or her preferences about such decisions—for example, 'Do not resuscitate' orders.

The physical examination in the geriatric patient: special considerations

A complete examination is required as usual, but think about the following areas as you go about obtaining the data.
1. **General assessment**
   - Check for postural blood pressure change.
   - Assess hydration, which may be impaired in older patients with cognitive dysfunction.
   - Look at the skin carefully for pressure sores or evidence of bruises from falls or elder abuse. Look at the skin for any evidence of skin cancer.
   - Measure weight and height to calculate the body mass index, as weight loss is common in the elderly.

2. **Heart**
   - If a systolic murmur is heard, consider whether this may be aortic stenosis, which, if severe, is likely to require treatment.
   - Ankle swelling may indicate venous insufficiency or antihypertensive drug use (e.g. calcium antagonists) rather than congestive cardiac failure. Ischaemic heart disease is common but often silent in the elderly.
3. **Chest**
   - Shortness of breath may be due to lung disease or cardiac disease, and these often coexist in the elderly.
4. **Gastrointestinal system**
   - Look at the dentition and check for dry mouth, which may impair eating.
   - The abdominal aorta may be palpable in the thin elderly patient. This may be falsely interpreted as an aneurysm, but if the aorta seems significantly enlarged, an aortic aneurysm needs to be excluded. If the aneurysm is leaking, the classical presentation includes back pain, abdominal distension, shock and poor asymmetrical peripheral pulses in the legs.
   - In patients with constipation from hard stool a mass may be felt in the left lower quadrant: this will clear with treatment for the constipation.
   - Perform a rectal examination and rule out faecal impaction, particularly if there is a history of faecal or urinary incontinence.
   - In patients with acute urinary retention an enlarged bladder may be felt: this problem can present with delirium.
5. **Nervous system**
   - Evaluation of mental status should be routine in geriatric patients. The mini-mental state examination is useful here.
   - Check for primitive reflex such as the glabellar tap, palmar mental reflex and grasp reflex, which are found in the elderly and may be evidence of dementia.
   - Test gait with the 'get up and go' test. Ask the patient to stand up out of a chair, walk 3 metres, turn around 180°, return to the chair and sit down.
6. **Eyes and ears**
   - Check vision and hearing as these may impair independent living.
7. **Rheumatological system**
   - Examine for deformities and functional disabilities, including the feet.
8. **Breasts**
   - Perform a breast examination in women, as the incidence of breast cancer greatly increases with age.

chapter 14

Assessment of the acutely ill patient

Acute disease; any disease which is attended with an increased velocity of blood, and terminates in a few days.

S Johnson, *A Dictionary of the English Language* (1755)

During your training, you will be expected to become expert in basic cardiac life support and advanced cardiac life support, and this training must be refreshed regularly.

If you come across an obviously very ill patient, the first step is to ask: 'Are you okay?' If the patient is **unresponsive** on gentle shaking, check whether the airway is patent and whether he or she is breathing, and then assess the circulation. Start cardiopulmonary resuscitation if the patient is not breathing or has no pulse, and try to send someone else to call for help.

If the patient is clearly **responding appropriately** to questions, and has skin that is normal in colour as well as being warm and dry, he or she is much less likely to need urgent intervention before appropriate history taking and a full physical examination can be done.

Gather key data as summarised by the mnemonic, AMPLE:

- **A**llergies
- **M**edication currently being taken and most recent medications taken
- **P**ast medical history
- **L**ast meal
- **E**vents preceding the current incident

If the patient is **tachypnoeic**, check pulse oximetry and start oxygen therapy unless there is a known contraindication.

If the patient is **bradycardic** or **tachycardic**, check the blood pressure and obtain an electrocardiogram (ECG).

If the patient is **hypotensive**, consider an intravenous fluid challenge, and measure the heart rate, blood pressure, respiratory rate and hourly urinary output (if necessary by placing a urinary catheter). Assess capillary refill time by depressing the patient's fingernail or toenail until it blanches and record the time it takes for the colour to become normal again, which is usually less than 2 seconds. A delayed capillary refill time occurs in hypovolemic or cardiogenic shock.

Examine the patient's chest for any obvious evidence of **tension pneumothorax** (characterised by increased breath sounds over the side of the tension pneumothorax, shift of the heart away from the tension pneumothorax, palpable subcutaneous emphysema and greatly distended neck veins). Assess the patient for possible **cardiac tamponade** (which can present with distended neck veins as well as low blood pressure and pulsus paradoxus). Examine the patient for any evidence of obvious bleeding or other trauma. Measure the patient's temperature. If this is elevated, consider taking blood and urine cultures.

If the patient's **level of consciousness becomes impaired** during your assessment, recheck the airway, breathing and circulation (ABCs), check the serum glucose (you must not miss hypoglycaemia) and obtain intravenous access immediately.

Assess level of consciousness using the AVPU system:
- **A**lert (normal)
- **V**erbal stimulus responsive
- **P**ainful stimulus responsive
- **U**nresponsive.

If the patient **responds only to a painful stimulus** or is **unresponsive**, assess the patient using the Glasgow coma scale (see box below).

Glasgow coma scale

Add up the scores for 1, 2 and 3: a total score of 4 or less = very poor prognosis for recovery; a total score > 11 = good prognosis for recovery.

1	Eyes	Open	Spontaneously 4
			To loud verbal command 3
			To pain 2
			No response 1
2	Best motor response	To verbal command	Obeys 6
		To painful stimuli	Localises pain 5
			Flexion—withdrawal 4
			Abnormal flexion posturing 3
			Extension posturing 2
			No response 1
3	Best verbal response		Oriented 5
			Confused, disoriented 4
			Inappropriate words 3
			Incomprehensible sounds 2
			None 1

Emergency care OSCE: hints panel

This man has had episodes of sudden loss of consciousness. Please examine him.

(a) Assess his level of consciousness, and test orientation in time, place and person.

(b) Examine his gait, then limbs and cranial nerves, looking for focal neurological signs (stroke, intracranial tumour).

(c) Note whether there are tongue lacerations (seizures).

(d) Auscultate for carotid bruits (carotid stenosis).

(e) Take his pulse (arrhythmias including atrial fibrillation or heart block) and blood pressure lying and sitting (postural hypotension).

(f) Examine the praecordium (signs of new murmurs, tamponade).

(g) Take his temperature and assess for neck stiffness (sepsis, meningism).

(h) Synthesise and present your findings.

chapter **15**

Examining the systems of the body

Medicine is an art, and attends to the nature and constitution of the patient, and has principles of action and reason in each case.

Plato (427–347 BC)

You need to be thoroughly familiar with a method for examining the various systems of the body. For example, a patient who presents with symptoms of heart disease needs to be examined for the peripheral signs of heart disease as well as for abnormalities of the heart itself. A systematic approach is essential, or signs of disease will be missed. A suggested method for the examination of the main systems is summarised in this chapter. Note that joint examination, examination of the relevant endocrine glands, and examination of the eyes, ears, nose and throat are directed at the affected parts of the body based on the history, and will not be summarised in this chapter.

The cardiovascular system (see Fig 15.1)

1. Arrange for the patient to lie at 45° and make sure the patient's chest and neck are fully exposed. Cover the breasts of a female patient with a towel or loose garment. Stand on the right side of the bed.
2. Stand back and inspect for **dyspnoea**, **cyanosis** (central or peripheral blue discolouration of the mucous membranes or skin), **jaundice** (yellow discolouration of the skin and sclerae) and **cachexia** (generalised muscle wasting, which may be a result of cardiac failure).
3. Pick up the patient's right hand, then left. Inspect the nails for **clubbing**. Also look for the peripheral stigmata of infective endocarditis: **splinter haemorrhages** are common (and are also caused by trauma). Look quickly, but carefully, at each nail bed, otherwise it is easy to miss splinters. Note any **tendon xanthomata** (hyperlipidaemia). Time the pulse at the wrist for **rate** and **rhythm**. Feel for **radiofemoral delay**

(which occurs in coarctation of the aorta). Pulse character is best assessed at the carotids.

4. Measure the patient's **blood pressure** with the patient lying down. An initial high reading may necessitate retaking it after the patient has spent 5 or 10 minutes calming down. If there are symptoms of postural dizziness or loss of blood is suspected, the blood pressure should also be measured while the patient stands (to assess for postural hypotension).

5. Look at the patient's eyes again for **jaundice** (e.g. due to haemolysis caused by a prosthetic valve) or **conjunctival pallor** (anaemia) and eyelid **xanthelasma** (hyperlipidaemia). You may also notice the classic **mitral facies** (bluish-red malar discolouration of mitral stenosis). Then inspect the mouth, using a torch, for the state of the **teeth** and **gums** (risk of endocarditis). Look at the tongue or lips for central **cyanosis**.

6. Assess the **jugular venous pressure** in the neck for height and character and the presence of **a waves** and **v waves**. Use the right internal jugular vein for this evaluation. This vein runs in the line between the angle of the jaw and the suprasternal notch. Look for a paradoxical rise with inspiration (Kussmaul's sign). Feel each **carotid pulse** separately. Assess the pulse character.

7. **The praecordium.** (1) *Inspection.* Look for **scars, deformity**, the site of the apex beat and **visible pulsations**. (2) *Palpation.* Feel for the position of the **apex beat**. Count down the correct number of interspaces. The normal position is the fifth left intercostal space, 1 cm medial to the mid-clavicular line. The **character** of the apex beat should be noted (**pressure-loaded, volume-loaded, dyskinetic, tapping** or **double** or triple apical impulse). Feel for an apical thrill and, if it is present, time it (systolic or diastolic or both). Palpate with the heel of your hand for a left **parasternal impulse** (which indicates right ventricular enlargement or left atrial enlargement) and for thrills. Feel at the base of the heart for a **palpable pulmonary component** of the second heart sound (P2) and for aortic thrills. Percussion is unnecessary. (3) *Auscultation.* Begin in the mitral area with first the bell and then the diaphragm. Listen for each component of the cardiac cycle separately.

8. Identify the **first** and **second heart sounds** and decide whether they are of normal intensity and whether the second heart sound is normally split. Listen for **extra heart sounds** and for **murmurs**. More than one abnormality may be present. Repeat the approach at the left sternal edge and then the base of the heart (aortic and pulmonary areas). Time each part of the cycle with the carotid pulse. If a murmur is present, work out its timing and loudness and the effect of dynamic manoeuvres on it.

9. Reposition the patient. First put the patient in the left lateral position. Again feel the apex beat for **character** (particularly tapping) and auscultate. Sit the patient up and palpate for **thrills** (with the patient in full expiration) at the left sternal edge and base. Then listen in those areas, particularly for aortic regurgitation.

10. Percuss the back of the patient's chest to exclude a **pleural effusion** (e.g. due to **left ventricular failure**) and auscultate for **inspiratory**

crackles (left ventricular failure). If there is a radiofemoral delay, also listen for a coarctation murmur over the back. Feel for **sacral oedema**.

11. Next lay the patient flat and examine the abdomen properly for **hepatomegaly** (e.g. from **right ventricular failure**) and a **pulsatile liver** (**tricuspid regurgitation**). Feel for **splenomegaly** (e.g. endocarditis) and an **aortic aneurysm**. Palpate both femoral arteries and auscultate here for bruits.

12. Examine all the **peripheral pulses** (popliteal, dorsalis pedis and posterior tibial). Look for signs of **peripheral vascular disease**, peripheral **oedema**, clubbing of the toes, Achilles tendon **xanthomata** and stigmata of infective endocarditis.

13. Examine the urine for **haematuria** (e.g. endocarditis).

14. Examine the fundi for **hypertensive** changes, and **Roth's spots** (endocarditis).

15. Take the patient's **temperature** (e.g. endocarditis or other infection).

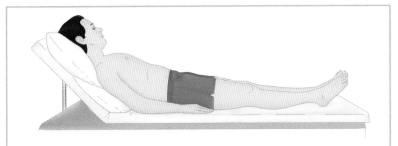

Lay the patient at 45° and make sure the patient's head and neck are fully exposed.

General inspection
  Marfan's syndrome, Turner's syndrome, Down syndrome
  Rheumatological disorders, e.g. ankylosing spondylitis (aortic regurgitation)
  Dyspnoea
  Cyanosis
  Jaundice
  Cachexia

Hands
  Radial pulses—right and left
  Radiofemoral delay
  Clubbing
  Signs of infective endocarditis— splinter haemorrhages
  Peripheral cyanosis
  Xanthomata

Blood pressure

Face
  Eyes
  • Sclerae—pallor, jaundice
  • Xanthelasma
  • Malar flush (mitral stenosis, pulmonary stenosis)
  Mouth
  • Cyanosis
  • Palate (high arched—Marfan's)
  • Dentition
Neck
  Jugular venous pressure
  • Central venous pressure height
  • Wave form (especially large v waves)
  • Carotids—pulse character

Figure 15.1 Examining the cardiovascular system   *continued*

Praecordium
Inspect
- Scars—whole chest, back
- Deformity
- Apex beat—position, character
- Abnormal pulsations
Palpate
- Apex beat—position, character
- Thrills
- Abnormal impulses
Auscultate
Heart sounds
Murmurs
Position patient
- Left lateral position
- Sitting forward (forced expiratory apnoea)
NB: Palpate for thrills again after positioning
Dynamic auscultation
- Respiratory phases
- Valsalva
Back (sitting forward)
Scars, deformity

Sacral oedema
Pleural effusion (percuss)
Left ventricular failure (auscultate)
Abdomen (lying flat—1 pillow only)
Palpate liver (pulsatile etc), spleen, aorta
Percuss for ascites (right heart failure)
Femoral arteries—palpate, auscultate
Legs
Peripheral pulses
Cyanosis, cold limbs, trophic changes, ulceration (peripheral vascular disease)
Oedema
Xanthomata
Calf tenderness
Clubbing of toes
Other
Urine analysis (infective endocarditis)
Fundi (endocarditis)
Temperature chart (endocarditis)

Figure 15.1 Examining the cardiovascular system *continued*

The respiratory system (see Fig 15.2)

1. Position the patient undressed to the waist and sitting over the side of the bed. Cover a woman's breasts with a towel or gown.
2. Inspect, while standing back, for **tachypnoea** at rest and any obvious asymmetry of movement. Count the **respiratory rate**. Look for the use of the **accessory muscles** of respiration, and any intercostal indrawing of the lower rib spaces anteriorly (an important sign of emphysema). Cachexia should also be noted (e.g. malignancy). Look around the room for the all-important **sputum mug** and ask to see its contents (e.g. for haemoptysis).
3. Pick up the patient's hands. Look for **clubbing**, peripheral **cyanosis**, **nicotine (tar) staining** and **pallor** of the palmar creases suggesting anaemia. Note any **wasting** of the small muscles of the hands (e.g. lung cancer involving the brachial plexus). Palpate the **wrists** for **tenderness** (hypertrophic pulmonary osteoarthropathy). Examine for a **flapping tremor** seen in carbon dioxide narcosis and liver failure.
4. Inspect the patient's face. Look closely at the eyes for **constriction** of the **pupils** and ptosis (Horner's syndrome from an apical lung cancer). Inspect the **tongue** for **central cyanosis**.

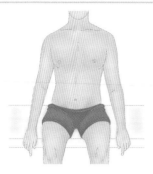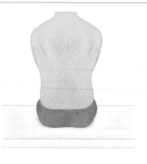

Position the patient sitting over the side of the bed.

General inspection
  Type of cough
  Rate and depth of respiration, and
    breathing pattern at rest
  Accessory muscles of respiration
  Sputum mug contents (blood, pus)
Hands
  Clubbing
  Cyanosis (peripheral)
  Nicotine staining
  Wasting, weakness—finger
    abduction and adduction (lung
    cancer involving the brachial
    plexus)
  Wrist tenderness (hypertrophic
    pulmonary osteoarthropathy)
  Pulse (tachycardia; pulsus
    paradoxus)
  Flapping tremor (CO_2 narcosis)
Face
  Eyes—Horner's syndrome (apical
    lung cancer), anaemia
  Mouth—central cyanosis
Trachea
  Voice—hoarseness (recurrent
    laryngeal nerve palsy)
Chest posteriorly
  Inspect
  • Shape of chest and spine
  • Scars
  • Prominent veins (determine
    direction of flow)
  Palpate
  • Cervical lymph nodes
  • Expansion
  • Vocal fremitus

  Percuss
  • Supraclavicular region
  • Back of chest
  • Axillae
  Auscultate
  • Breath sounds
  • Adventitious sounds
  • Vocal resonance
Chest anteriorly
  Inspect
  • Radiotherapy marks, other signs as
    noted above
  Palpate
  • Supraclavicular nodes
  • Expansion
  • Vocal fremitus
  • Apex beat
  Percuss
  Auscultate
  Pemberton's sign (superior vena
    cava obstruction)
Cardiovascular system (lying at 45°)
  Jugular venous pressure (superior
    vena cava obstruction)
  Cor pulmonale
Forced expiratory time
Other
  Lower limbs—oedema, cyanosis
  Temperature chart (infection)
  Evidence of malignancy or pleural
    effusion: examine the breasts, liver,
    rectum, all lymph nodes

Figure 15.2 Examining the respiratory system

5. Palpate the position of the trachea. If the **trachea** is displaced, concentrate on the upper lobes for physical signs. Also note the presence of a **tracheal tug** (downward movement of the trachea with each inspiration, which indicates severe airflow obstruction). Ask the patient to speak (note **hoarseness**, which may be caused by recurrent laryngeal nerve palsy) and then cough, and note whether this is a loose cough, a dry cough or a bovine cough.

6. Examine the patient's **chest**. You may wish to examine the front first, or go to the back to start. The advantage of the latter is that there are often more signs there, unless the trachea is obviously displaced.

7. If you start at the back, inspect the **spine**. Look for kyphoscoliosis and any signs of ankylosing spondylitis (which may cause decreased chest expansion and upper lobe fibrosis). Look for thoracotomy **scars**.

8. Palpate the **cervical nodes** from behind. Then examine for expansion— first **upper lobe expansion**, which is best assessed by looking over the patient's shoulders at clavicular movement during moderate respiration. The affected side will show a delay or decreased movement. Then examine **lower lobe expansion** by palpation. Note **asymmetry** and reduction of movement.

9. Ask the patient to bring the elbows together in the front to move the scapulae out of the way. Examine for **vocal fremitus**, then percuss the back of the chest.

10. Auscultate the back of the chest. Note **breath sounds** (whether **normal** or **bronchial**) and their intensity (**normal** or **reduced**). Listen for **adventitious sounds** (**crackles** and **wheezes**). Finally examine for **vocal resonance**. If a localised abnormality is found, try to determine the abnormal lobe and segment.

11. Return to the front of the chest. Inspect again for chest deformity, **radiotherapy changes** and **scars**. Palpate the **supraclavicular nodes**. Then proceed with percussion and auscultation as before. Listen high up in the axillae too. Before leaving the chest feel the axillary nodes and examine the breasts. Test for **Pemberton's sign**.

12. Lay the patient down at 45° and measure the **jugular venous pressure**. Then examine the **praecordium** for signs of pulmonary hypertension (**cor pulmonale**: a prominent parasternal impulse, a loud pulmonary component of the second heart sound, and sometimes a right ventricular third or fourth heart sound and a murmur of tricuspid regurgitation).

13. Examine the **liver** (e.g. palpable because of ptosis or metastatic cancer, or pulsatile due to tricuspid regurgitation).

14. Take the patient's **temperature**.

The gastrointestinal system (see Fig 15.3)

1. Position the patient correctly with one pillow for the head and the abdomen completely exposed.

2. Look, while standing back, at the general appearance and for obvious signs of chronic liver disease.

3. Pick up the patient's hands. Ask the patient to extend his or her arms and hands and look for **asterixis**. Look also at the nails for **clubbing** and for **liver (white) nails**. Note the presence of **palmar erythema** or **Dupuytren's contractures**.

4. Look at the arms for **bruising**, **scratch marks**, **spider naevi** and proximal muscle wasting.

5. Go to the face. Note any scleral changes (e.g. **jaundice**, **anaemia**) or **iritis**. Feel for parotid enlargement, then inspect the mouth with a torch and spatula for **angular stomatitis**. Smell the breath for **fetor hepaticus**.

6. Look at the chest for **spider naevi**, and in men for **gynaecomastia** and loss of body hair.

7. Inspect the abdomen from the side, squatting to the patient's level. Large masses may be visible. Ask the patient to take slow deep breaths and look for the outlines of the liver, spleen and gall bladder. If distended, note whether this is central, peripheral or in one flank.

8. Palpate lightly in each region for **masses**, having asked first whether any area is particularly tender. This will avoid causing pain and may provide a clue to sites of possible pathology. Next palpate more deeply in each region, then feel specifically for **hepatomegaly** and **splenomegaly**. If there is hepatomegaly, confirm this with percussion and estimate the span (normal < 13 cm). This procedure is repeated for splenomegaly. Always roll the patient onto the right side and palpate again if the spleen is not felt at first. Attempt now to feel the kidneys bimanually.

9. Percuss for **ascites**. If the abdomen is resonant right out to the flanks, do not roll the patient over. Otherwise test for **shifting dullness**.

10. By auscultation note the presence of **bowel sounds**. Listen also for **bruits**, **hums** and **rubs**. Always auscultate over the liver, spleen or kidneys if these are enlarged or palpable, or over any palpable **mass**.

11. Examine the groin. Palpate for **inguinal lymphadenopathy**. Examine for **hernias** by asking the patient to stand and then cough. The **testes** must be palpated.

12. Now look at the legs for **oedema** and **bruising**. Neurological examination of the legs may be indicated if there are signs of chronic liver disease (e.g. from alcohol abuse).

13. If the liver is **enlarged** or cirrhosis is suspected, the patient should be sat up to 45° and the jugular venous pressure estimated (to exclude right heart failure as a cause of liver disease).

14. While the patient is sitting up, palpate in the **supraclavicular fossae** for lymph nodes and feel over the lower back for **sacral oedema**. If ascites is present, it is necessary to examine the chest for pleural effusions. If malignant disease is suspected, examine all the lymph node groups, the breasts and the lungs.

15. A **rectal examination** should be performed and specimens of the patient's vomitus or faeces should be inspected, if available.

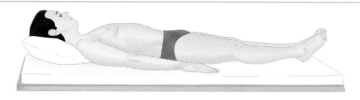

Position the patient lying flat on the bed with one pillow for the head and the abdomen completely exposed.

General inspection
Jaundice (liver disease)
Pigmentation (haemochromotosis, Whipple's disease)
Xanthomata (chronic cholestasis)
Mental state (encephalopathy)

Hands
Nails
• Clubbing
• Leuconychia
Palmar erythema
Dupuytren's contractures (alcohol)
Arthropathy
Hepatic flap

Arms
Spider naevi
Bruising
Wasting
Scratch marks (chronic cholestasis)

Face
Eyes
• Sclera: jaundice, anaemia, iritis
Parotids (alcohol)
Mouth
• Breath: fetor hepaticus
• Lips: stomatitis, leucoplakia, ulceration, localised pigmentation (Peutz–Jeghers syndrome), telangiectasia (hereditary haemorrhagic telangiectasia)
• Gums: gingivitis, bleeding, hypertrophy, pigmentation, monilia
• Tongue: atrophic glossitis, leucoplakia, ulceration

Cervical/axillary lymph nodes

Chest
Gynaecomastia
Spider naevi
Body hair loss

Abdomen
Inspect
• Scars
• Distension
• Prominent veins—determine direction of flow (caput medusae; inferior vena cava obstruction)
• Striae
• Bruising
• Pigmentation
• Localised masses
• Visible peristalsis
Palpate
• Superficial palpation—tenderness, rigidity, outline of any mass
• Deep palpation—organomegaly (liver, spleen, kidney), abnormal masses
Roll on to right side (spleen)
Percuss
• Viscera outline
• Ascites—shifting dullness
Auscultate
• Bowel sounds
• Bruits, hums
• Rubs

Groin
Genitalia
Lymph nodes
Hernial orifices (standing up)

Legs
Bruising
Oedema
Neurological signs (alcohol)

Other
Rectal examination—inspect (fistulae, tags, blood, mucus), palpate (masses)
Urine analysis (bile)
Cardiovascular system (jugular venous pressure, signs of right heart failure if hepatomegaly)
Temperature chart (infection)

Figure 15.3 Examining the gastrointestinal system

The genitourinary system (see Fig 15.4)

1. Lay the patient flat on the bed while making the usual general inspection. Note particularly the patient's mental state and whether the patient has a sallow complexion, the state of **hydration** and whether the patient is **hiccupping** or **hyperventilating** (possible signs of renal failure).
2. Pick up the patient's hands and look at the nails for **leuconychia** or white transverse lines that may occur in hypoalbuminaemia (e.g. nephrotic syndrome).
3. Examine the patient's wrists and arms for vascular access sites. Assess the patency of an **arteriovenous fistula** by palpating for a thrill. Get the patient to hold out his or her hands and look for **asterixis**. Then inspect the patient's arms for **subcutaneous nodules** (e.g. calcium phosphate deposits), bruising, pigmentation and scratch marks (chronic renal failure).
4. Go on to the face and begin by examining the eyes for **anaemia** (chronic renal failure). Examine the mouth for **dryness** (dehydration) or **fetor**.

Position the patient lying flat on the bed.

General inspection
Mental state
Hyperventilation (acidosis) hiccups
Hydration
Subcutaneous nodules (calcium phosphate deposits)

Hands
Nails—leuconychia; white transverse lines; single white band; distal nail brown, proximal nail white or pink (half and half nails)

Arms
Bruising
Pigmentation
Scratch marks
Myopathy

Face
Eyes—anaemia, jaundice, band keratopathy
Mouth—dryness, ulcers, fetor
Rash (vasculitis)

Abdomen
Scars—dialysis, operations
Kidneys—transplant kidney
Bladder
Liver
Lymph nodes
Ascites
Rectal examination (prostatomegaly)

Back
Tenderness
Oedema

Chest
Heart—pericarditis, failure
Lungs—infection, pulmonary oedema

Legs
Oedema—nephrotic syndrome, cardiac failure
Bruising
Pigmentation
Scratch marks
Neuropathy
Vascular access

Urine analysis
Specific gravity, pH
Glucose—diabetes mellitus
Blood—nephritis, infection, stone
Protein—nephritis, nephrotic syndrome

Other
Blood pressure—lying and standing
Fundoscopy—hypertensive and diabetic changes

Figure 15.4 Examining the genitourinary system

Note the presence of any vasculitic rash on the face. Note any neck scars (e.g. parathyroid surgery).

5. Lie the patient flat and examine the abdomen. Look for **scars** indicating peritoneal dialysis or operations including a **renal transplant**. Then examine the liver and spleen (enlargement may occur in polycystic disease). Palpate for enlarged **kidneys by ballottement.** Feel for the presence of an **abdominal aortic aneurysm**. Percuss over the bladder to detect enlargement. Listen for aortic and renal bruits.

6. Sit the patient up and palpate the back for tenderness and sacral oedema.

7. Look at the **jugular venous pressure** with the patient at 45°. Examine the heart for signs of pericarditis, pericardial effusion or cardiac failure and the lungs for pulmonary oedema.

8. Lay the patient down again. Look at the legs for **oedema** (due to the **nephrotic syndrome** or **cardiac failure**), bruising, pigmentation, scratch marks or the presence of gout. Examine for **peripheral neuropathy** (decreased sensation, loss of reflexes in chronic renal failure).

9. Measure the **blood pressure** with the patient lying and then standing (for **orthostatic** (postural) **hypotension**) and perform **fundoscopy** to look for hypertensive or diabetic changes.

10. Perform a rectal examination, if indicated, to feel for **prostatomegaly**.

11. Finally, perform **urinalysis**, testing for specific gravity, pH, glucose, blood, protein and leucocytes.

The haematological system (see Fig 15.5)

1. Position the patient as for a gastrointestinal examination and make sure he or she is fully undressed.

2. Look for **bruising, pigmentation, cyanosis, jaundice** and **scratch marks** (suggesting pruritis due to myeloproliferative disease or lymphoma). Look for frontal bossing and note the racial origin of the patient (e.g. in thalassaemia).

3. Pick up the patient's hands. Look at the **nails** for **koilonychia** (spoon-shaped nails—iron deficiency) and the changes of **vasculitis**. Pale palmar creases may indicate **anaemia**. Evidence of **arthropathy** may be important (e.g. **rheumatoid arthritis** and **Felty's syndrome**, recurrent **haemarthroses** in bleeding disorders, secondary **gout** in myeloproliferative disorders).

4. Examine the **epitrochlear** nodes.

5. Note any bruising on the arms. Remember **petechiae** are pinhead haemorrhages, while **ecchymoses** are larger bruises. Palpable purpura indicates a vasculitis.

6. Go to the axillae and palpate the **axillary** nodes. There are five main areas: **central, lateral** (above and lateral), **pectoral** (most medial), **infraclavicular** (apical) and **subscapular** (most inferior).

7. Look at the face. Inspect the eyes, note jaundice, pallor or haemorrhage of the sclerae, and the injected sclerae of **polycythaemia**.

Position the patient lying flat on the bed with one pillow for the head.

General inspection
Bruising (thrombocytopenia, scurvy, haemophilia)
• Petechia (pinhead bleeding)
• Ecchymoses (large bruises)
Pigmentation (lymphoma)
Rashes and infiltrative lesions (lymphoma)
Ulceration (neutropenia)
Cyanosis (polycythaemia)
Plethora (polycythaemia)
Jaundice (haemolysis)
Scratch marks (myeloproliferative diseases, lymphoma)
Racial origin
Pallor (anaemia)
Hands
Nails—koilonychia
Palmar crease pallor (anaemia)
Arthropathy (haemophilia, secondary gout, drug treatment)
Epitrochlear nodes
Axillary nodes
Face
Sclera—jaundice, pallor, conjunctival suffusion (polycythaemia)
Mouth—gum hypertrophy (monocytic leukaemia), ulceration, infection, haemorrhage (marrow aplasia); atrophic glossitis, angular stomatitis (iron, vitamin deficiencies)

Cervical nodes (sitting up)
Palpate from behind
Bony tenderness
Spine
Sternum
Clavicles
Shoulders
Abdomen (lying flat) and genitalia
Organomegaly (spleen, liver)
Legs
Vasculitis (Henoch-Schönlein purpura—buttocks, thighs)
Bruising
Pigmentation
Ulceration (e.g. haemoglobinopathies)
Neurological signs (subacute combined degeneration in vitamin B_{12} deficiency, peripheral neuropathy)
Other
Fundi (haemorrhages, infection)
Temperature chart (infection)
Urine analysis (haematuria, bile)
Rectal and pelvic examination (blood loss)

Figure 15.5 Examining the haematological system

8. Examine the mouth. Note gum **hypertrophy** (e.g. from acute monocytic leukaemia or scurvy), ulceration, infection, haemorrhage, **atrophic glossitis** (e.g. from iron deficiency, or vitamin B_{12} or folate deficiency) and angular stomatitis. Look for tonsillar and adenoid enlargement (e.g. leukaemia).
9. Sit the patient up. Examine the cervical nodes from behind: **submental, submandibular, jugular** chain, **posterior triangle, postauricular, preauricular** and **occipital**. Then feel the **supraclavicular** area from the front.
10. Tap the **spine** with your fist for **bony tenderness** (which may be caused by an enlarging marrow—e.g. in myeloma or carcinoma). Press gently on the sternum, clavicles and shoulders for bony tenderness.
11. Lay the patient flat again. Examine the abdomen. Note any hepatomegaly. Don't forget to feel the testes. Consider performing a rectal (and pelvic

examination) for evidence of bleeding. Spring the hips for pelvic tenderness.

12. Examine the legs. Note particularly **leg ulcers** (e.g. due to haemolytic anaemia, thalassaemia, Felty's syndrome and polycythaemia). Examine the legs from a **neurological** aspect, for peripheral neuropathy (e.g. vitamin B_{12} deficiency, which also causes posterior column loss and upper motor neuron signs).

13. Examine the **fundi**, look at the **temperature** chart and test the **urine**.

The nervous system (see Figs 15.6–15.8)

1. **Handedness, orientation and speech.** Ask the patient whether he or she is right- or left-handed. As a screening assessment, ask for the patient's name, the present location and the date. Next ask the patient to name an object pointed at and then ask the patient to point to a named object in the room (to test for dysphasia). Ask the patient to say 'British constitution' (to test for dysarthria).

2. **Neck stiffness and Kernig's sign.** If the symptom onset is acute, look for these signs of meningism.

3. **Cranial nerves.** The patient should be sat over the edge of the bed, if possible. Begin with a general inspection of the head and neck, looking for craniotomy scars, neurofibromas, facial asymmetry, ptosis, proptosis, skew deviation of the eyes or pupil inequality.

   - **The second nerve.** Test visual acuity with the patient wearing his or her spectacles. Test each eye separately, while the other is covered with a small card.

     Examine the visual fields by confrontation, using a hatpin. If visual acuity is very poor, map the fields using your fingers. Look into the fundi.

   - **The third, fourth and sixth nerves.** Look at the pupils, noting the shape, relative sizes and any associated **ptosis**. Use a pocket torch and shine the light from the side to gauge the reaction of the pupils to light. Assess both the **direct** and **consensual** responses. Test **accommodation** by asking the patient to look into the distance and then at the hatpin placed about 20 cm from the nose.

     Assess **eye movements** with both eyes first, getting the patient to follow the pin in each direction. Ask about **diplopia**. Look for **failure of movement** and for **nystagmus**.

   - **The fifth nerve.** Test the **corneal reflexes** gently and ask the patient whether the touch of the cottonwool on the cornea can be felt. The sensory component of this reflex is the fifth nerve and the motor component is the seventh nerve.

     Test **facial sensation** in the three divisions: **ophthalmic**, **maxillary** and **mandibular**. Test **pain** sensation with a new pin and map any area of sensory loss from dull to sharp. Test light touch as well so that **sensory dissociation** can be detected, if present.

     Examine the motor division of the fifth nerve by asking the patient to **clench the teeth** while you feel the masseter muscles. Then get

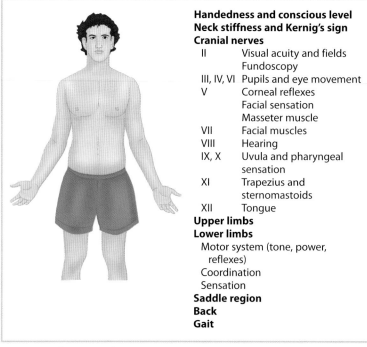

Handedness and conscious level
Neck stiffness and Kernig's sign
Cranial nerves

II	Visual acuity and fields
	Fundoscopy
III, IV, VI	Pupils and eye movement
V	Corneal reflexes
	Facial sensation
	Masseter muscle
VII	Facial muscles
VIII	Hearing
IX, X	Uvula and pharyngeal sensation
XI	Trapezius and sternomastoids
XII	Tongue

Upper limbs
Lower limbs
  Motor system (tone, power, reflexes)
  Coordination
  Sensation
Saddle region
Back
Gait

Figure 15.6 Examining the nervous system

the patient to open his or her mouth while you attempt to force it closed. A unilateral lesion causes the **jaw to deviate** towards the weak (affected) side.

Test the **jaw jerk**. With the patient's mouth open, tap with a tendon hammer one of your own fingers placed on the patient's chin. Brisk closure of the mouth occurs in an upper motor neuron lesion.

- **The seventh nerve.** Test the muscles of facial expression. Ask the patient to look up and **wrinkle the forehead**. Look for loss of wrinkling and feel the muscle strength by pushing down on each side. Next ask the patient to **shut his or her eyes** tightly and compare the two sides. Tell the patient to **grin** and compare the nasolabial grooves.
- **The eighth nerve.** Whisper a number 60 cm away from each of the patient's ears. Perform **Rinné's** and **Weber's** tests with a 256 Hz tuning fork if there is deafness. Examine the external auditory canals and the eardrums, if this is indicated.
- **The ninth and tenth nerves.** Look at the palate and note any **uvular** displacement. Ask the patient to say 'ah' and look for symmetrical movement of the soft palate (tenth). Test gently for **pharyngeal sensation** (the ninth nerve is the sensory component and the tenth nerve the motor component if a gag reflex occurs). Ask the patient to speak to assess hoarseness, and to cough and swallow.

- **The eleventh nerve.** Ask the patient to shrug his or her shoulders, and feel the **trapezius** while pushing the shoulders down. Then ask the patient to turn his or her head against resistance, and also feel the bulk of the **sternomastoid**.
- **The twelfth nerve.** While examining the patient's mouth, inspect the tongue for wasting and fasciculation. Next ask the patient to protrude the tongue. Unilateral paralysis results in **deviation of the tongue** towards the paralysed side.

Then examine the skull and auscultate for carotid bruits.

4. **Upper limbs** (see Fig 15.7). Ask the patient to sit over the side of the bed facing you.

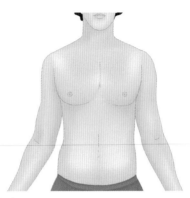

Figure 15.7 Upper limbs

- Examine the **motor system** systematically every time. Inspect first for wasting and fasciculations.
- Ask the patient to hold out both hands with the arms extended and to close the eyes. Look for **drifting** of one or both arms (caused by an upper motor neuron weakness, a cerebellar lesion or posterior column loss).
- Also note any **tremor**, or **pseudoathetosis** due to proprioceptive loss. Feel the **muscle bulk** and note any muscle tenderness.
- Test **tone** at the wrists and elbows by passively moving the joints at varying velocities.
- Assess **power** at the shoulders, elbows, wrists and fingers.
- If indicated, test for an ulnar nerve lesion (Froment's sign) and a median nerve lesion (pen-touching test).
- Examine the **reflexes**: biceps (C5, C6), triceps (C7, C8), brachioradialis (C5, C6) and finger jerks (C8).
- Assess **coordination** with finger–nose testing and look for dysdiadochokinesis and rebound.
- Examine the **sensory system** after motor testing because this can be time-consuming. First test the **spinothalamic pathway** (pain). Start proximally and test each dermatome. Next test the **posterior column**

pathway. Use a 128 Hz tuning fork to assess **vibration** sense. Place the vibrating fork on a distal interphalangeal joint initially.

- Examine **proprioception** with the distal interphalangeal joint of the index finger.
- Test **light touch** with cottonwool. Touch the skin lightly (do not stroke) in each dermatome.
- Feel for thickened nerves—the ulnar at the elbow, the median at the wrist and the radial at the wrist—and feel the axillae if there is evidence of a proximal lesion. Note any scars, and finally examine the neck, if relevant.

5. **Lower limbs** (see Fig 15.8(a)).
   - Test the **stance** and **gait** first, if possible. Ask the patient to walk normally for a few metres and then turn around quickly and walk back. Then ask the patient to walk heel-to-toe to exclude a mid-line cerebellar lesion. Ask the patient to walk on the toes (an S1 lesion will make this impossible) and then on the heels (an L4 or L5 lesion causing footdrop will make this impossible). Look for shuffling (Parkinson's disease), hemiplegia (the foot is swung in an arc and remains plantarflexed) or a wide-based gait (cerebellar disease).

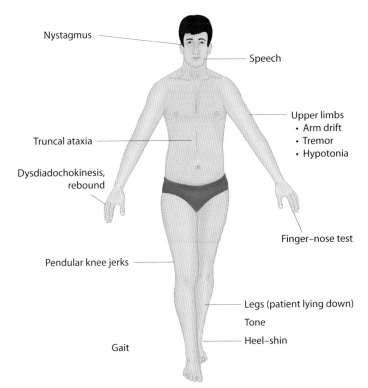

Figure 15.8 Lower limbs: **(a)** walking

continued

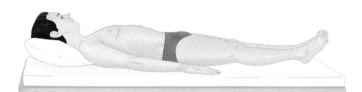

Figure 15.8 Lower limbs: **(b)** supine *continued*

- Ask the patient to lie on the bed with his or her legs entirely exposed (Fig 15.8(b)). Note any **fasciculations**. Feel the **muscle bulk** of the quadriceps and run your hand up each shin, feeling for wasting of the anterior tibial muscles.
- Test **tone** at the knees and ankles. Test **clonus** at the knee and ankle.
- Assess **power** at the hips, knees and ankles.
- Elicit the **reflexes**: knee (L3, L4), ankle (S1, S2) and plantar response (L5, S1, S2).
- Test **coordination** with the heel–shin test, toe–finger test and tapping of the feet.
- Examine the **sensory system** as for the upper limbs: pinprick, then vibration and proprioception (beginning with the big toe), and then light touch. If there is sensory loss involving the whole leg or legs, attempt to establish a sensory level on the trunk and abdomen. Examine **sensation in the saddle region** and test the **anal reflex** (S2, S3, S4).
- Look for deformity, scars and neurofibromas on the patient's back. Palpate for tenderness over the vertebral bodies and auscultate for bruits. Perform the **straight leg raising test**.

chapter 16

Writing and presenting the history and physical examination

Study sickness while you are well.
Thomas Fuller (1608–1661)

Writing up the history and physical examination

The written entries in a patient's notes are an important legal document. The notes may be used for reference throughout the admission and during any future admissions to hospital. The initial admitting notes are usually the most comprehensive. A system for recording these is outlined below. The exact format, however, will be different for different types of admissions. The routine admission of a young person for a minor surgical procedure under local anaesthetic will be much less detailed than the admission of an elderly patient with a complicated medical problem.

Further entries to the notes usually record ward rounds and decisions by the treating team about investigations and treatment.

If a patient becomes acutely ill on the ward, a record must be made of the details of the problem, the examination findings, the proposed investigations and their results, and the advice of the senior staff that have been consulted. The entry must be updated frequently if the patient's condition changes.

The history
Personal information

Record the patient's name, gender and date of birth. Write down the date and time of the examination.

Presenting (principal) symptoms (PS)

A short sentence identifies the major presenting complaints and their duration; it is useful to quote the patient's own words.

215

History of present illness (HPI)

Do not record every detail; rather, prepare short prose paragraphs or use dot points telling the story of the illness in chronological order (from the past to the present time). Describe the characteristics of each symptom. Note why the patient presents at this time. Also describe any past medical problems that are related to the current symptoms. Include the relevant positive and negative findings on the systems review here.

If there are many seemingly unrelated problems, summarise these in an introductory paragraph and present the history of each problem in a separate paragraph. List the patient's current medications and doses, the indications for their use (if they are known) and any side effects. Record your impression of the reliability of the historian and, if the patient was unable to give the history, describe who the source was.

Past history (PH)

List in chronological order past medical problems and surgical operations, and past medication use, if relevant. Record any history of allergy (particularly drug allergy). A history of blood transfusions should be noted.

Social history (SH)

Describe as a minimum the patient's occupation, marital status and recent travel. Smoking habits, alcohol use, analgesic use and other non-medical drug use should also be described.

Family history (FH)

Describe causes of mortality or relevant morbidity in the patient's first-degree relatives and, if indicated, draw a family tree.

Systems review (SR)

All directly relevant information should be incorporated into the HPI or PH.

The physical examination (PE)

Under each of the major systems, list the relevant positives and negatives using brief statements. Begin with the system most relevant to the presenting symptoms.

Provisional diagnosis, problem list and plans

Using a sentence or two, summarise the most important findings and then give a provisional diagnosis (PD) and list the differential diagnosis (DD).

List all the active problems that require management. Outline the diagnostic tests and therapy planned for each problem. Sign your name and then print your name and position underneath.

An example of a medical history

Personal details: Mr W Witheridge, age 72, retired botanist.

Presenting symptoms: 3 weeks of progressive exertional dyspnoea with 2 days of dyspnoea at rest.

History of present illness

- Two nights of severe orthopnoea; unable to sleep except briefly while sitting in a chair.
- Mild exertional shortness of breath for nearly 10 years.
- He is unable to walk 50 metres on the flat.
- No associated chest tightness or pain.
- No wheeze or cough.
- No fever.
- No recent change in medications.
- No asthma or known lung disease. No other relevant positive symptoms on systems review.

Cardiac history

Previous myocardial infarction 5 years ago, treated with thrombolytic drugs. No known valvular heart disease or history of rheumatic fever.

Smoked 25 cigarettes a day until the time of his infarct—30 packet years.

Risk factors for heart disease

Total cholesterol 6.7 mmol/L, a family history of ischaemic heart disease—his 55-year-old brother had hypertension for 30 years—inadequate control. Salt intake high, drinks 3–4 litres of fluid a day. Alcohol—25 g a week. There is no history of diabetes mellitus. Only occasional non-steroidal anti-inflammatory drugs.

Other symptoms

10 years of nocturia three times per night. He denies other urinary tract symptoms.

Current medications

Aspirin, 100 mg daily; and metoprolol (a beta-blocker), 100 mg twice a day.

Past history

- Gastric ulceration 3 years ago—successfully treated with a 14-day course of antibiotics and a proton pump inhibitor; no recurrence of symptoms. Appendectomy and tonsillectomy in his youth.
- He has no drug allergies that he knows of and has never required a blood transfusion.

Social history

- Lives in retirement with his wife, who is well.
- Interests; gardening, history of medicinal plants, no other hobbies. No pets.
- No recent overseas travel or long car trips. No use of over-the-counter medications.

Family history

His father died of a myocardial infarct at age 64 years, and his mother died of colon cancer at age 84 years. Both sons (42 and 39 years) are alive and well. No other relevant family history.

Physical examination

Breathless and uncomfortable at rest. Respiratory rate—24 breaths/minute.

continued

Cardiovascular
- No cyanosis. No clubbing. No splinter haemorrhages.
- Pulse rate 90 beats/minute and regular.
- Blood pressure 180/110 mmHg, lying and standing.
- Temperature 37 °C.
- JVP not elevated.
- Apex beat 2 cm displaced, dyskinetic.
- Heart sounds (HS): S1 (first) and S2 (second) present and normal, S3 (third) present.
- Pansystolic murmur grade 3/6 maximum at the apex consistent with mitral regurgitation.

Chest
- Trachea in the mid-line.
- Expansion normal right and left.
- Normal percussion note bilaterally.
- Bilateral medium basal mid-inspiratory crackles and occasional expiratory wheeze over the right and left lung fields. No areas of bronchial breathing.

Abdomen
- Well-healed appendix scar present.
- Abdomen soft, no tenderness.
- Liver not palpable, no other masses (spleen, kidneys).
- No ascites.
- Normal bowel sounds.
- Rectal examination deferred (the patient was too unwell at the time of admission).

Legs—no calf tenderness. No peripheral oedema. Peripheral pulses present and equal. No visible varicose veins.

Central nervous system (CNS)—alert and orientated. No neck stiffness.

Cranial nerves (assessed after initial treatment)

II—acuity and fields normal; fundi normal.

III, IV and VI—pupils equal, circular and concentric—react normally to light and accommodation; eye movements normal; no nystagmus.

V—sensation and motor function normal.

VII—muscles of facial expression normal.

VIII—hearing normal.

IX, X—no uvular displacement.

XI—normal power.

XII—no fasciculation or displacement of tongue.

Upper limbs

No wasting, fasciculations, tremor.

Tone normal.

Power normal (shoulders, elbows, wrists, fingers).

Reflexes normal and symmetrical	Right	Left
Biceps	++	++
Triceps	++	++
Brachioradialis	++	++

Coordination normal.

Sensation—pain, proprioception normal.

Lower limbs
Gait normal.
No wasting.
Tone normal; no clonus.
Power normal (hips, knees, ankles).
Reflexes normal and symmetrical

	Right	Left
Knee	++	++
Ankle	++	++
Plantars	↓	↓

Coordination normal.
Sensation—pain, proprioception normal.
Provisional diagnosis: left ventricular failure secondary to ischaemic heart disease.
Differential diagnosis: angina, pulmonary embolus, chronic obstructive pulmonary disease.
Investigations:
   Electrocardiogram
   Chest X-ray
   Full blood count
   Electrolytes, creatinine, liver function tests
   Echocardiogram
Comment
The aetiology of his cardiac failure is most likely to be ischaemic heart disease (previous infarct) or hypertensive. He has signs of mitral regurgitation, which may be secondary to cardiac failure or, less likely, the cause. There is no known history of chronic lung disease, although he has been a chronic smoker. The history and examination are not very suggestive of pulmonary embolism.

Presenting the history and physical examination

It is not enough to take a history, examine a patient and make a diagnosis. You must also be able to pass this information on by means of written notes and case presentations to colleagues and others involved in the patient's care.

Presenting a patient's history and physical examination in the long case exam

The presentation of a patient's history and physical examination to examiners (a long case exam) is a very formal exercise. An effective approach is to begin by giving the examiners some information about the patient's age and sex, and then to explain whether it is a diagnostic problem or a treatment problem, or both. For example, you might say: 'I am presenting Mrs X, a 75-year-old woman with a diagnostic and management problem of the sudden onset of left-sided weakness.' This lets the examiners know that you have thought about the problem and are not just presenting a series of facts. The presentation should continue starting with more detail about the presenting symptoms. It is important not to bore the examiners with long lists of irrelevant negative findings, but to have this information available if asked for it. At the end of your presentation you should present a differential diagnosis (in order of likelihood) and a proposed plan of investigation and treatment (management).

Presenting a patient's history and physical examination to a consultant

The long case format is not the best way to present a patient's details to a senior colleague, especially in the middle of the night. There are three reasons for contacting a consultant about a new patient:

1. A polite call to let the consultant know about a stable patient. Some consultants want to know about new patients at any time, while others are happy to be told when it is convenient (e.g. after grand rounds are over, at a reasonable hour of the morning or when a series of routine admissions has been saved up).
2. A call to seek advice and discuss the proposed management of a complicated patient.
3. A call to ask the consultant to come in to see the patient or to perform a procedure.

The reason for the call should be given at the start of the conversation. Consultants are rarely interested in a patient's family history or in hearing a long list of irrelevant negative findings. The appropriate course is to give a brief history of the presenting problem and objective findings, followed by a differential diagnosis and management plan. Then stop talking to allow for discussion or approval of the plan.

Presenting a patient's history and physical examination at a handover meeting

Here the patient is being presented to colleagues who will be taking over the management of the patient. These meetings vary in formality. It is essential that patients who are unwell or have unresolved problems be discussed in the greatest detail. The team taking over care of the patient needs to know where the patient is, some biographical details about the patient, and briefly the presenting clinical features and provisional diagnosis.

Investigations that are available must be outlined and those that have been ordered but are not yet available identified so that these results are not missed. A sick patient may need urgent and frequent review by the new team.

If consultants or senior registrars are present, their advice should be sought about more difficult patients.

Often a particular patient is chosen for more detailed discussion as a teaching exercise. This patient's history and examination findings may have to be outlined in relatively more detail, but not to the point of a long case presentation.

List of OSCEs

Final remarks

He has been a doctor a year now and has had two patients, no, three, I think—yes, it was three; I attended their funerals.

Samuel Clemens (Mark Twain) (1835–1910)

Medical education is not completed at the Medical school; it is only begun.

William H Welch (1850–1934)

You should now be well on your way in your journey towards acquiring the vital clinical skills of history taking and physical examination. Despite the increasing acceleration of technological innovation in the medical field, these are the skills that you will utilise throughout your medical career. Of course, the journey will never end, because learning and relearning these skills is a lifelong occupation.

Good luck!

Further reading

Apley AG, Solomon L. *Physical examination in orthopaedics*. London: Hodder Education; 1997.

Baker T, Nikolic G, O'Connor S. *Practical cardiology*. 2nd edn. Sydney: Elsevier; 2008.

Browse NL. *An introduction to the symptoms and signs of surgical disease*. 4th edn. New York: Oxford University Press; 2005.

Douglas G, Nicol F, Robertson C. *Macleod's clinical examination*. 11th edn. Edinburgh: Churchill Livingstone; 2005.

Enelow AJ, Forde DL, Brummel-Smith K. *Interviewing and patient care*. 4th edn. Melbourne: Oxford University Press; 1996.

Fuller G. *Neurological examination made easy*. 4th edn. Edinburgh: Churchill Livingstone; 2008.

Lloyd M, Bor R. *Communication skills for medicine*. 2nd edn. London: Churchill Livingstone; 2004.

McGee S. *Evidence-based physical diagnosis*. 2nd edn. Philadelphia: WB Saunders; 2007.

Talley NJ, O'Connor S. *Clinical examination. A systematic guide to physical diagnosis*. 5th edn. Sydney: Elsevier; 2006.

Talley NJ, O'Connor S. *Examination medicine: A guide to physician training*. 5th edn. Sydney: Elsevier; 2006.

Talley NJ, Segal I, Weltman MD. *Gastroenterology and hepatology: A clinical handbook*. Sydney: Elsevier; 2008.

Tierney LM, Henderson MC. *The patient history. Evidence-based approach*. New York: McGraw-Hill; 2005.

Index

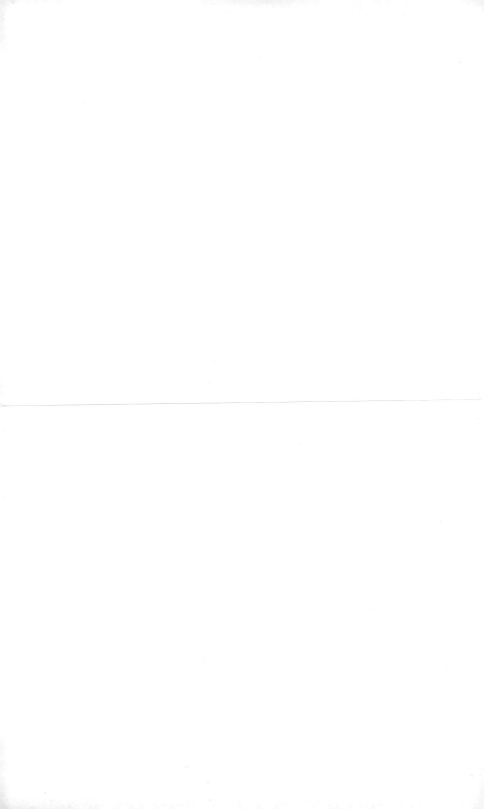